Study Guide for

Fundamentals of

Nursing

Care

Concepts,
Connections,
& Skills

SECOND EDITION

Study Guide for

Fundamentals of
Nursing
Care

Concepts, Connections, & Skills

SECOND EDITION

Marti A. Burton, RN, BS
Curriculum Developer
Instructor, Link to Nursing Program
Canadian Valley Technology Center
Yukon, Oklahoma

Linda J. May Ludwig, RN, BS, MEd
Retired Nursing Instructor
Canadian Valley Technology Center
El Reno, Oklahoma

F.A. Davis Company • Philadelphia

F. A. Davis Company
1915 Arch Street
Philadelphia, PA 19103
www.fadavis.com

Printed in the United States of America

Last digit indicates print number: 10 9 8 7 6 5 4 3 2

Senior Acquisitions Editor: Thomas Ciavarella
Director of Content Development: Darlene D. Pedersen
Content Project Manager II: Victoria White
Art & Design Manager: Carolyn O'Brien

As new scientific information becomes available through basic and clinical research, recommended treatments and drug therapies undergo changes. The author(s) and publisher have done everything possible to make this book accurate, up to date, and in accord with accepted standards at the time of publication. The author(s), editors, and publisher are not responsible for errors or omissions or for consequences from application of the book, and make no warranty, expressed or implied, in regard to the contents of the book. Any practice described in this book should be applied by the reader in accordance with professional standards of care used in regard to the unique circumstances that may apply in each situation. The reader is advised always to check product information (package inserts) for changes and new information regarding dose and contraindications before administering any drug. Caution is especially urged when using new or infrequently ordered drugs.

ISBN: 978-0-8036-3975-1

To the Students Who Use this Workbook

Our purpose in writing this student workbook is to help you capture the important information from each chapter and be able to apply it to situations you will likely encounter as a nursing student and a nurse.

Because people learn in different ways, we urge you to identify the way you learn best, whether it is by hearing, by seeing and reading, or by touching and doing. You will need to learn the essential information in each chapter in a way that works best for you.

Suggestions for auditory learners—those who learn best by hearing—include:

- Review information by speaking it aloud.
- Repeat information aloud to help you memorize or comprehend.
- Explain the information to another person.
- Watch videos of skills while listening to a narrator.
- Read your text reading assignment aloud into a small recorder; play it back for more audio learning.
- After you feel you can thoroughly answer all of your objectives, write the answers down; then read the answers into the recorder for additional playback and audio learning.
- Get together with peers in small groups and quiz each other aloud.

Suggestions for visual learners—those who learn best by seeing—include:

- Color-code information with highlighters, using different colors for different types of information.
- Write out explanations for difficult concepts in your own words.
- Use sticky notes with keywords and concepts placed where you will see them frequently.
- Watch videos of skills being performed step by step.

Suggestions for kinesthetic learners—those who learn best by touching and doing—include:

- Take notes, draw pictures, and make charts as you study and listen.
- Make flashcards with definitions or explanations on one side and a word or concept on the other side; study by flipping the cards and identifying what is on the other side.

- Write key concepts on different colored flashcards; then sort the cards according to category, topic, or similarities to help you learn how to connect the information.
- Make models of the organs from clay or paper to learn the structures of a body system.
- Watch and listen to videos of skills, using the ability to stop and start the skill after each step; obtain various supplies that will be demonstrated in the videos; study and manipulate them concurrently with the skills video.

This workbook is designed in sections to help you learn one aspect of the chapter at a time. These sections include:

Key Terms Review—Matching and fill-in-the-blank questions help you learn new terminology.

Connection Questions—Multiple-choice and short answer questions help you understand and apply information presented in the connection features. These include clinical applications, anatomy and physiology, delegation and supervision, laboratory and diagnostic tests, home health and long-term care settings, patient teaching, and real-world illustrations.

Review Questions—Multiple-choice, matching, true/false, and short answer questions cover the important information in the chapter. *Note that multiple-choice questions often have more than one correct answer, so read carefully and thoughtfully, then mark all answers that apply. This helps prepare you for the multiple answer questions on the NCLEX.*

Application and Critical Thinking Questions—Multiple-choice, scenarios, and brief answer questions help you pull together the information in the chapter and apply it to situations you may often encounter as a student nurse or as a nurse.

Documentation Exercise—Scenario(s) describe patient care that you will then document on the appropriate chart forms, just as you would in patient care.

Every section of the workbook is designed to help you learn and apply critical concepts so you will be prepared to care for your patients. We want you to be not just nurses, but good nurses who think critically about their patients.

Marti Burton and Linda Ludwig

Contents

Introduction to Nursing

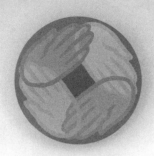

The Vista of Nursing

Name: _____

Date: _____

Course: _____

Instructor: _____

Part 1. Key Terms Review

Match the following Key Term(s) or italicized words from your text with the correct description.

_____ 1. Licensed practical or vocational nurse (LPN/LVN)

_____ 2. Associate degree nurse (ADN)

_____ 3. Nurse Practice Act

_____ 4. Health Occupations Students of America (HOSA)

_____ 5. Scope of practice

_____ 6. Quality and Safety Education for Nurses (QSEN)

_____ 7. Evidence-based practice

a. The law in each state that governs nurses' actions; addresses each level of nursing

b. A national organization specifically for students in health occupations educational programs; membership is open to both high-school and adult students

c. Most basic of all the entry-level options for nurses with full-time programs lasting from 9 months to 1 year

d. Limitations and allowances of what can be done as a nurse

e. Entry-level education of registered nurses; minimum of 2 years at a community college

f. Problem-solving approach using best evidence from nursing research studies, patient data, and patient's preferences and values

g. Project that focuses on knowledge, skills, and attitudes needed by nurses to continually improve the quality and safety of patient care

Fill in the blank with the correct Key Term(s) or italicized words from your text.

8. When students in ADN, diploma, and BSN programs complete all coursework and graduate, they are eligible to take the _____, and after they pass it, they become registered nurses.

9. Nurses who are educated in hospital-based nursing education programs, of which there are few, are referred to as _____ nurses.

10. When students in an LPN or LVN program complete their educational program, they will take the

    _____, and after they

    pass it, they become licensed practical or licensed

    vocational nurses.

11. The professional organization for licensed practical/

    vocational nurses is the _____

    _____

    _____.

12. Nurses who complete their nursing education at a

    university, earning a 4-year college degree, are

    _____ nurses.

Part 2. Connection Questions

Choose the correct answer(s). In some questions, more than one answer is correct. Select all that apply.

13. The purpose(s) of the Clinical Connections in this book is/are to help you
    a. understand the chapter better through a detailed case study.
    b. identify actions to take and information to consider when caring for patients.
    c. understand your thoughts and feelings about caring for specific types of patients.
    d. connect what you read in this book with what you will see and do during clinical experiences.

14. Which of the following are concerns when you are providing care for elderly patients?
    a. These patients have difficulty expressing their concerns.
    b. These patients often have chronic illnesses, sensory deficits, and multiple medications.
    c. These patients are most often cared for in their own homes or the homes of relatives.
    d. These patients are most often cared for in long-term care facilities.

15. When you care for pediatric patients, you must keep in mind that they
    a. often have multiple medical problems.
    b. have difficulty understanding what is happening and expressing their feelings during procedures.
    c. often have no previous experience to prepare them for illness or treatment, so they are frightened.
    d. are cared for in a physician's office or clinic, rather than a hospital.

16. A unique aspect of home health is that
    a. the patients are not actually sick but more in need of education and information.
    b. many family members are available to help you when you perform a procedure.
    c. fewer supplies and less equipment are available than in a hospital setting.
    d. the nurse is alone in the home with no other health-care staff to help make decisions about care.

17. Which of the following is true of working in long-term care?
    a. The setting is more homelike.
    b. You will care only for people who are confused.
    c. You will need to use an easy, calming approach to residents.
    d. Changes in behavior can indicate health problems in the elderly.

18. Which are your responsibilities as a nursing student regarding laboratory and diagnostic test results?
    a. You do not have any responsibility because this is the physician's responsibility.
    b. Check the test results often and note any abnormal findings.
    c. Notify the physician of significant abnormal results.
    d. Adjust medication orders based on abnormal results.

19. What might be the outcome if you delegate a task to unlicensed assistive personnel (UAP) or a certified nursing assistant (CNA) that is not within his or her scope of practice?
    a. You are liable for any poor outcomes, but the UAP is not liable.
    b. The charge nurse will take the blame for any errors made by the UAP.
    c. No harm can come to a patient based on delegation of tasks to the UAP.
    d. Both you and the UAP can be in legal jeopardy.

Write a brief answer to the following questions.

20. What is a common desire of successful nursing students?

_____

_____

_____

21. Explain the purpose of the Post-Conference Connection.

_____

_____

_____

Part 3. Review Questions

Choose the correct answer(s). In some questions, more than one answer is correct. Select all that apply.

22. Which is true of nursing care in hospitals during the 1700s and early 1800s?
    a. Nursing care was provided by family members and priests.
    b. Nursing care was provided by deaconesses.
    c. Nursing care was provided by the poor and lower classes.
    d. Nursing care was provided by female midwives only.

23. Kaiserswerth deaconesses were women who
    a. trained at the first school of nursing.
    b. went to various places to teach other women to be nurses.
    c. established the first nursing associations.
    d. were educated at the same school as Florence Nightingale.

24. When did laws requiring licensing of nurses first come into being?
    a. In the early 1800s
    b. In 1836
    c. In 1897
    d. In the early 1900s

25. Which nurse in history was known as the "Angel of the Battlefield" during the U.S. Civil War?
    a. Clara Barton
    b. Dorothea Dix
    c. Florence Nightingale
    d. Mary Mahoney

26. Which nurse in history established modern nursing and is famous for giving nursing care during the Crimean War?
    a. Clara Barton
    b. Dorothea Dix
    c. Florence Nightingale
    d. Mary Mahoney

27. Who was the first African American nurse in the United States?
    a. Linda Richards
    b. Lillian Wald
    c. Dorothea Dix
    d. Mary Mahoney

28. Which nurse in history developed the first nurse's notes and established the first school of nursing in Japan?
    a. Linda Richards
    b. Lillian Wald
    c. Isabel Hampton Robb
    d. Mary Mahoney

29. Which nurse in history was instrumental in establishing a 3-year training program for nurses and worked for licensure examinations and nursing registration?
    a. Linda Richards
    b. Lillian Wald
    c. Isabel Hampton Robb
    d. Mary Mahoney

30. Graduates of which program(s) take the NCLEX-RN?
    a. Baccalaureate degree nursing program
    b. Associate degree nursing program
    c. Diploma nursing program
    d. Licensed practical or vocational nursing program

31. Which is true of the Nurse Practice Acts in all states?
    a. LPNs/LVNs must practice under the supervision of an RN or physician.
    b. RNs must practice under the supervision of a physician.
    c. The act is enforced by each state's nursing board.
    d. The act establishes the scope of practice for each level of nursing practice.

32. Which are the responsibilities of the nurse?
    a. Caring for more than one patient at a time
    b. Helping families understand the care of the patient after discharge
    c. Determining the need for and ordering diagnostic tests
    d. Noticing changes in the patient's condition and notifying the appropriate health-care professional

33. Which is/are example(s) of unprofessional conduct that could result in the loss of a person's nursing license?
    a. Stealing from a patient while caring for him or her in the home
    b. Neglecting to ensure that a resident in a long-term care setting is receiving adequate food and fluids
    c. Caring for a patient while under the influence of alcohol
    d. Leaving a long-term care facility during an assigned shift so that nursing assistants are unsupervised
    e. Making an error when administering medications to a patient

34. Which student organization is connected with the American Nurses Association?
    a. NSNA
    b. NFLPN
    c. HOSA
    d. DECA

35. Which student organization holds competitions for medical-related skills?
    a. NSNA
    b. NFLPN
    c. HOSA
    d. DECA

36. Which focus of QSEN ties into providing individualized care of patients, including their preferences, values, and needs in their plan of care?
    a. Teamwork and collaboration
    b. Evidence-based practice
    c. Quality improvement
    d. Patient-centered care

Match the following nursing theorists to their theories.

_____37. Sister Callista Roy

_____38. Jean Watson

_____39. Madeleine M. Leininger

_____40. Dorothea Orem

a. Developed the self-care deficit theory, which explains what nursing care is required when people cannot care for themselves
b. Developed the adaptation model, inspired by the strength and resiliency of children; relates to the choices people make as they adapt to illness and wellness
c. Developed the caring theory, which focuses on nursing as an interpersonal process
d. Developed the culture care diversity and universality theory

Write a brief answer to the following questions.

41. What does a nursing theory include?

_____

_____

_____

_____

42. List three ways nurses coordinate the care of several patients during a shift.

_____

_____

_____

_____

Part 4. Application and Critical Thinking Questions

Write a brief answer to the following questions.

43. Although starting nursing school may be the realization of your goal, why is it only the beginning of setting and achieving your goals?

_____

_____

_____

_____

44. How is a licensed practical/vocational nurse different from an associate degree nurse in education and licensure?

_____

_____

_____

_____

45. As you begin nursing school, you are convinced that you want to be an obstetrical nurse. What will you expect in your education program regarding any specialization in nursing?

_____

_____

_____

_____

46. Why is it necessary for all nurses to continue to learn after completing their basic nursing education?

_____

_____

_____

_____

47. Explain how nursing can be both an art and a science.

_____

_____

_____

_____

48. Describe three attributes of a good and professional nurse.

_____

_____

_____

_____

49. Explain how nurses have more opportunities to influence the health of their patients than do other health-care professionals.

_____

_____

_____

_____

50. Explain how evidence-based practice will influence your practice as a nurse.

_____

_____

_____

_____

Choose the correct answer(s). In some questions, more than one answer is correct. Select all that apply.

51. While you are a nursing student, you make an error when giving your patient medications. The patient is not aware of the error and neither is your instructor. The incorrect medication could cause interactions with the patient's other medicines, but it might not cause any problems. What will you do?
    a. Wait to see whether the patient suffers any reactions or problems, then explain what happened.
    b. Tell the patient to notify only you if he or she experiences any unusual feelings or problems.
    c. Tell the patient what happened but ask him or her not to tell anyone because you will then get into trouble.
    d. Explain to your instructor what happened and follow facility protocol for reporting medication errors.
    e. Keep all information about the error to yourself. If the patient has a problem, the doctor can order another medication to counteract it.

Situation Questions

♦ *Scenario: Questions 52 and 53 refer to this scenario.*

A recent newspaper story in your town tells about a resident in a long-term care facility who was wheelchair bound. She was also somewhat confused. This elderly lady found her way to an open stairway door and fell down an entire flight of stairs in her wheelchair. She ended up dying from her injuries. The licensed nurse on duty that day is accused of not keeping the door closed as required by the fire marshal and safety inspectors. In addition, the nursing staff is accused of not supervising the resident closely and allowing harm to come to her.

52. Which example(s) of unprofessional conduct has this licensed nurse and the staff exhibited?
    a. Diversion of drugs from prescribed patient to personal use
    b. Failure to supervise nursing assistants and unlicensed assistive personnel adequately
    c. Failure to adequately care for patients or conform to minimum standards of nursing practice
    d. Criminal conduct

53. The licensed nurse in this situation could face disciplinary action by the Board of Nursing. What is the most severe outcome that could result from that disciplinary action?
    a. The nurse will lose his or her license.
    b. The nurse will be required to give safety talks to other nurses.
    c. The nurse will not be allowed to practice nursing for a minimum of 1 year.
    d. The nurse would not be able to supervise nursing assistants for a minimum of 1 year.

Documentation Exercise

Nurses must document all care that they give to patients. In addition, they must plan the care they will give and then evaluate the effectiveness of that care. You will learn how to do all of this in later chapters. In later workbook chapters, you will be asked to practice your documentation skills.

For this chapter, you will document your own education plan, rather than documenting about a patient. Just as you will plan patient care as a nurse, you need to plan your future in nursing. Use the following blank form as you develop your personal education plan. Write your name on the top line and today's date on the next line.

54. Write one to two paragraphs to answer the following questions:
    • When do you anticipate completing your basic nursing education? Give the month and the year.
    • What do you plan to do after graduation from nursing school? Will you work? If so, where do you plan to work?
    • If you do not plan to work as a nurse after graduating, what do you plan to do? If you are continuing your education, identify the school and program you plan to attend.
    • What do you see yourself doing 3 years from now? Explain why you see that in your near future.
    • What do you see yourself doing 5 years from now? Explain why you see that in your future.

Nursing Education Plan for:

_____

Date: _____

_____

_____

_____

_____

_____

_____

_____

_____

_____

_____

_____

_____

_____

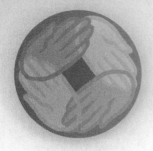

Health Care Delivery and Economics

Name: _____

Date: _____

Course: _____

Instructor: _____

Part 1. Key Terms Review

Match the following Key Term(s) or italicized words from your text with the correct description.

_____ 1. Medicare

_____ 2. Managed care

_____ 3. Case management

_____ 4. Medicaid

_____ 5. Third-party payer

_____ 6. Health maintenance organization

_____ 7. Diagnosis-related group

_____ 8. Preferred provider organization

_____ 9. Point of service

_____ 10. Primary care physician

a. Patient care approach aimed at coordinating the care of patients who are vulnerable, at risk, or cost intensive so that their specific needs are met in the most cost-effective manner while still bringing them to optimum health

b. A federally and state-funded health insurance program for individuals who are poor and medically indigent, pregnant women, individuals with disabilities, and children meeting income level requirements

c. The federal government's health insurance program for people older than 65 years or those with certain disabilities or conditions

d. The insurance company that finances health care provided to a beneficiary

e. A system of health-care delivery aimed at managing the cost and quality of access to health care

f. A type of insurance program where a primary care physician serves as gatekeeper, but the members are not capitated; insured people can seek care from physicians who are both in and out of the network

g. The gatekeeper for access to medical services

h. A cost-containment program featuring a primary care physician (PCP) as the gatekeeper to eliminate unnecessary testing and procedures

      i. A classification of illnesses and diseases that is then used to determine the amount of money paid to a hospital by Medicare

      j. A group of health-care providers who contract with a health insurance company to provide services to a specific group of patients on a discounted basis

Fill in the blank with the correct Key Term(s) or italicized words from your text.

11. When a person stays overnight or longer in a health-care facility, he or she is referred to as a(n)

_____.

12. _____ can be one or many types of health or medical services provided to patients in their home because they are confined to their home by an illness or disability.

13. _____ is a medically directed, nurse-coordinated program providing a continuum of home and inpatient care for the patient who is terminally ill and his or her family.

14. Empowering the patient to take control of and manage his or her care is called _____.

15. When patient care is provided by different individuals who perform tasks based on his or her skills, education, and licensure, it is called _____.

16. In _____ one nurse is responsible for all aspects of nursing care for his or her assigned patients.

17. When a primary care physician cannot successfully treat a patient's condition, he or she makes a(n)

_____ to a specialist.

18. When care is provided to a person without admitting him or her to a health-care facility, the person is referred to as a(n) _____.

19. A facility that specializes in intense physical, occupational, and speech therapy is called a(n) _____ facility.

Part 2. Connection Questions

Choose the correct answer(s). In some questions, more than one answer is correct. Select all that apply.

20. At what age are people eligible for Medicare?
    a. 62
    b. 63
    c. 64
    d. 65

21. Insurance companies will only pay costs when a procedure is deemed medically necessary. By medically necessary, they mean
    a. the procedure has to be a reasonable intervention, given the patient's diagnosis.
    b. the patient has to want to have the procedure done.
    c. the procedure has to treat an illness or injury.
    d. the procedure must contribute to the patient's sense of well-being.

22. A 58-year-old patient is in an ICU step-down unit at an acute care hospital after having a cerebrovascular accident (stroke) with right-sided weakness. He is medically stable but needs assistance with all activities of daily living (ADLs). The doctors think he may be able to regain all his former level of function. The appropriate level of care at this point in the patient's progress is a(n)
    a. acute care hospital.
    b. long-term acute care hospital (LTACH).
    c. skilled nursing facility (SNF).
    d. rehabilitation facility.

23. Which of the following is a criterion for admission to a skilled nursing facility?
    a. The patient has made maximum progress and is considered stable.
    b. The patient has been hospitalized within the last 30 days.
    c. The patient requires intensive physical therapy.
    d. The patient will not be able to return to independent living and will be a resident.

24. Which of the following can be considered a disadvantage of team nursing?
    a. Patients have more than one name to remember when asking for their nurse.
    b. Patients may not like different team members and ask to work with just one.
    c. Care can be fragmented unless there is good communication among team members.
    d. The team leader may delegate tasks that are inappropriate to a team member's level of expertise.

25. An LPN is the team leader for another LPN and certified nursing assistant, all of whom are caring for 10 patients in a long-term care facility. The second LPN applies a pressure ulcer dressing incorrectly. Which of the following is the best response for the team leader to make when she discovers the error?
    a. "You aren't performing this task correctly. Why don't you review the procedure manual to figure out what you did wrong?"
    b. "I see you tried to do a good job, but I am ultimately responsible for all the care given to our patients. If there are any other dressing changes required, let me know and I will do them."
    c. "You did a good job with this dressing change. I see one step here that you may have overlooked. Tell me how you did it so we can figure out if it was done according to the procedure."
    d. "It looks like you forgot a step here. Is something bothering you today, or do you just not understand the procedure?"

Write a brief answer to the following questions.

26. Explain why a team leader must have good communication skills.

_____

_____

_____

27. Explain why patients should know the details of their insurance plans.

_____

_____

_____

Part 3. Review Questions

Write a brief answer to the following question.

28. Give one reason why patients are cared for by a team of health-care professionals from different specialty areas.

_____

_____

_____

Choose the correct answer(s). In some questions, more than one answer is correct. Select all that apply.

29. Changes in health insurance coverage implemented in Phase 1 of the Affordable Care Act include:
    a. Some preventative services are available at no cost to the consumer.
    b. Children cannot be turned down due to pre-existing conditions.
    c. Young adults are able to stay on their parent's policy until age 30 years.
    d. There are no longer any "lifetime limits" of coverage.

Indicate whether the following statements about the Affordable Care Act are True (T) or False (F).

_____30. "Health Care Exchanges" are just another name for private insurance policies.

_____31. If a state opts out of the Health Care Exchanges, the citizens will then all be put on Medicaid.

_____32. As of January 1, 2014, everyone will be required to have health insurance or else pay a special tax.

_____33. One way the expenses of the Affordable Care Act will be paid for is by preventing Medicare reimbursement to hospitals from rising as fast as previously.

Match the health-care practitioner on the left to the appropriate functions on the right.

_____34. Nurse practitioner

_____35. Registered nurse

_____36. Licensed practical/ vocational nurse

_____37. Certified nursing assistant

_____38. Physician's assistant

_____39. Medical social worker

a. Practices within a defined scope under the supervision of a physician, dentist, or RN; provides direct patient care and supervises assistive personnel

b. Provides psychosocial support to patients, families, or vulnerable populations; advises caregivers; counsels patients; plans for patients' needs after discharge; and arranges for needed care such as home health

c. Performs patient care duties and assists nursing staff; performs more complicated tasks, including sterile procedures, in some states

d. Employed by physicians or hospitals to work closely with physician and assist in directing patient care

e. Certified in a specific area of practice; carries an advanced practice license and can diagnose illnesses, prescribe medications, and order treatments

f. Practices nursing within a defined scope under the direction of a physician; provides direct patient care, manages departments, and supervises other nurses and assistive personnel

Fill in the blank with the correct health-care practitioner.

40. The personnel who help patients with disabilities to develop new skills, recover lost skills, or maintain functional skills so that they can perform activities of daily living (ADLs) are called _____.

41. The personnel who help diagnose swallowing difficulties are called _____.

Choose the correct answer(s). In some questions, more than one answer is correct. Select all that apply.

42. What are the two most important factors in economic decisions about patient care?
    a. Appropriate level of care and health insurance plan
    b. Medical necessity and appropriate level of care
    c. Medical necessity and type of health insurance
    d. Type of health insurance and expected length of hospitalization

43. Health care provided by various companies and purchased by the individual or an employer is called
    a. Medicare.
    b. Medicaid.
    c. managed care.
    d. private insurance.

44. One important consideration in managing costs is making sure the patient is placed in which of the following?
    a. Appropriate level of care
    b. Managed care
    c. A health maintenance organization (HMO)
    d. Acute care hospital

45. Which of the following is the major difference between an assisted living facility and an independent living facility?
    a. There is no major difference.
    b. Independent living facilities do not provide nursing care.
    c. Residents must have medical needs to be placed in an assisted living facility.
    d. Assisted living facilities provide activities, but independent living facilities do not.

46. An 81-year-old woman had a total hip replacement 1 month ago but has had difficulty swallowing related to an injury from the breathing tube. Three weeks ago she had a feeding tube placed through her abdominal wall directly into her stomach (a gastrostomy) to help her get enough calories and for administering medications. She has been improving and has just started a thickened-liquids diet. Which of the following would be the appropriate level of care for her?
    a. Acute care hospital
    b. Skilled nursing facility
    c. Rehabilitation facility
    d. Long-term acute care hospital

Write a brief answer to the following question.

47. Describe three types of rehabilitation facilities.

_____

_____

_____

_____

Choose the correct answer(s). In some questions, more than one answer is correct. Select all that apply.

48. A 48-year-old male patient has been hospitalized for 6 weeks in an acute care facility after being involved in a car accident. He was driving while intoxicated and admitted to being an alcoholic. He went through alcohol withdrawal while he was recovering from his injuries and has received some information about alcoholism treatment from a psychologist. He has his own business, is married, has four children, and has adequate health insurance. What care options are best for this man at this time?
    a. Inpatient drug and alcohol rehabilitation facility
    b. Ambulatory care clinic
    c. Outpatient mental health services
    d. Home health care

49. Which of the following represents the desired outcomes of cardiac rehabilitation?
    a. Prevent worsening heart disease, new cardiac events, and premature death
    b. Provide exercise and nutritional guidance
    c. Provide care in a more cost-effective manner
    d. Help patients recover as quickly as possible

50. Which of the following statements are true regarding health departments?
    a. They are funded by all levels of government.
    b. They provide immunizations.
    c. They track and treat communicable diseases.
    d. They run the Women, Infants, and Children (WIC) health program.

51. What is the role of the social worker in home health care?
    a. Provides psychosocial support
    b. Helps families prepare for the patient's needs after discharge
    c. Provides dressing changes and determines ongoing need for treatment
    d. Arranges for community services such as Meals on Wheels or transportation to and from office visits

52. Which of the following represents a benefit of home health care?
    a. Allows people to stay in their own homes instead of being in a facility
    b. Prevents fragmentation of care
    c. Is more cost effective than inpatient care
    d. Prevents complications

53. Which of the following services can be provided through home health care?
    a. Infusion therapy
    b. Occupational therapy
    c. Physical therapy
    d. Wound therapy

54. For Medicare to pay for home health services, which of the following two criteria must be met?
    a. Skilled services required; patient is homebound
    b. Nursing care only is required; patient is homebound
    c. Nonskilled services required; patient is not necessarily homebound
    d. Physical, occupational, or speech therapy required; patient is not necessarily homebound

55. Although there is no hard and fast rule, when is the appropriate time to initiate hospice care?
    a. Patient is expected to live less than 3 months
    b. Patient is expected to live 6 months or less
    c. Patient is expected to live less than 1 year
    d. At the time the patient is diagnosed with a terminal illness regardless of life expectancy

56. The National Hospice Organization's definition of hospice states that hospice
    a. provides a continuum of home and inpatient care.
    b. is coordinated by nurses.
    c. cares for the patient and family.
    d. does not include pain medication management.

Indicate whether the following statements are True (T) or False (F).

57. _____ Fragmentation of care is more likely to occur with team nursing than with primary nursing.

58. _____ Delegation skills are helpful when leading a nursing care team but not essential because each team member knows his or her level of expertise.

59. _____ Team leaders probably know more about each patient in his or her care because they have other staff to help them.

60. _____ As a member of a nursing care team, but not the leader, it is important for a nurse to have good communication skills.

61. _____ In client-centered care, patients are encouraged to have a voice in goal setting and in deciding how the goals will be met.

62. _____ In client-centered care, the nurse makes sure other members of the health-care team such as the phlebotomist, EKG technician, and respiratory therapist perform their tasks in a timely manner.

63. _____ Cross-training of staff is more important in primary care than it is in client-centered care.

64. _____ Primary care nursing means that one nurse does all the care for one patient.

65. _____ Primary care works best on general care floors, not intensive care units (ICUs).

66. _____ Primary care must be performed by an RN.

67. _____ The main goal of case management is to make sure patients at high risk get the care they need at the least cost to the facility.

68. _____ The nurse case manager usually provides direct, hands-on care.

69. _____ A case manager's main function is to coordinate and facilitate the care of several different patients concurrently.

Fill in the blanks with the appropriate term or terms.

70. _____ is a government-run insurance plan for people older than a certain age.

71. _____ is a government-run insurance program for poor people and some people who are disabled.

72. Blue Cross/Blue Shield, Aetna, and Prudential are examples of _____ insurance programs.

73. A primary care physician acting as a gatekeeper to eliminate unnecessary testing and procedures is a feature of a _____.

Choose the correct answer(s). In some questions, more than one answer is correct. Select all that apply.

74. Diagnosis-related groups (DRGs) are classifications of illnesses or procedures used to
   a. perform quality-of-care research.
   b. identify patients at high risk who will benefit from case management.
   c. determine appropriate level of care.
   d. standardize the amount the government will pay for a specific illness.

75. TRICARE for retired military personnel and their families and CHAMPVA for veterans are examples of
   a. preferred provider organizations (PPOs).
   b. point of service (POS) insurance plans.
   c. insurance for special populations.
   d. insurance through charitable organizations.

Part 4. Application and Critical Thinking Questions

Write a brief answer to the following questions.

76. You work in an acute care facility that is considering designating one wing of your floor for patients who have no insurance or have Medicaid. Decide whether this is a good idea and explain why you do or do not think so.

_____

_____

_____

_____

_____

_____

_____

_____

77. Give an example of fragmentation of care that could result when a team nursing model for care delivery is used.

_____

_____

_____

_____

_____

78. Explain how you, as a team leader for an LPN/LVN and a UAP with 10 patients, would create a system for ensuring good communication about the patients.

_____

_____

_____

_____

_____

79. Explain how a patient's insurance plan might affect his or her care. Focus on a patient with Medicaid versus a patient with high-quality private insurance.

_____

_____

_____

_____

_____

Documentation Exercise

For this chapter, you will document your preferred nursing care delivery model and why you think this model will be best. Use the following blank form. Write your name on the top line and today's date on the next line.

80. Write one to two paragraphs to answer the following questions:
    - Which nursing model appeals to you?
    - Which model do you think will provide the best patient care and why?
    - Which model will provide the most job satisfaction?
    - What do you see as potential weak points in the model and how would you address them?

Name: _____

Date: _____

_____

_____

_____

_____

_____

_____

_____

_____

_____

_____

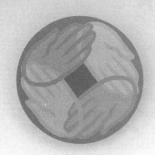

Nursing Ethics and Law

Name:	_____
Date:	_____
Course:	_____
Instructor:	_____

Part 1. Key Terms Review

Match the following Key Term(s) or italicized words from your text with the correct description.

_____ 1. Abandonment

_____ 2. Assault

_____ 3. Battery

_____ 4. Ethics

_____ 5. Negligence

_____ 6. Empathy

_____ 7. Nurse Practice Act

_____ 8. NCLEX

_____ 9. Advocate

_____10. Scope of practice

_____11. Malpractice

a. Values that influence your behavior

b. To stand up for the patient's best interest

c. Ability to intellectually understand another's feelings

d. Provides protection to a voluntary caregiver at accident sites

e. Legal boundaries for nursing care

f. Nurse's action fails to meet standard of care and results in patient injury

g. Premature cessation of patient care without adequate notice

h. To intentionally harm a patient

i. Showing intent to touch a patient without permission

j. Nurse licensing examination

k. Patient injury resulting from nurse's failure to meet responsibility to the patient

l. Provides scope of practice in each state

m. Ability to feel sorry for another person

Part 2. Connection Questions

Choose the correct answer(s). In some questions, more than one answer is correct. Select all that apply.

12. Who owns a hospitalized patient's medical record?
    a. The patient
    b. The physician
    c. The hospital
    d. The patient's primary care nurse
    e. The patient's insurance company

13. Which of the following nursing actions would be considered proactive prevention of lawsuits?
    a. Meeting your patient's needs
    b. Treating your patient with dignity
    c. Developing good nurse–patient rapport
    d. Keeping conversation with your patient to a minimum to reduce chances of offending the patient
    e. Explaining procedures and ensuring the patient's understanding before performing the procedure

14. Your patient has been newly diagnosed with AIDS. You are good friends with the patient's wife and feel that you should tell her so that she can be tested. Which of the following statement(s) is (are) true?
    a. Because the wife is considered an immediate family member, it is permissible for you to discuss the patient's test results with her.
    b. Failure to disclose the serious diagnosis to the wife could be considered negligence.
    c. The patient must give permission for the AIDS test results to be disclosed to the wife.
    d. Discussing the test results without the patient's permission is a breach of HIPAA.

Write a brief answer to the following question.

15. Can it still be considered breach of patient confidentiality if the patient information was *accidentally* overheard by a visitor sitting at the table behind you in the cafeteria?

_____

Part 3. Review Questions

Write a brief answer to the following questions.

16. Which type of hospital in the United States forbids that copies of patient chart documents be carried outside the hospital walls, even if the patient's name and identifying data are cut off the document?

_____

_____

_____

17. Which health-care provider is identified as the patient's advocate?

_____

_____

_____

18. In a court of law, there is a standard regarding documentation in patients' records. What is this standard and what does it mean?

_____

_____

_____

_____

19. Explain how to legally correct an error a nurse makes in documentation.

_____

_____

_____

_____

20. Documenting something that you did not actually do would be legally considered as what?

_____

Choose the correct answer(s). In some questions, more than one answer is correct. Select all that apply.

21. A 17-year-old girl would be considered an emancipated minor in which of the following situations or conditions?
    a. Marriage
    b. Has lived alone and supported herself for 15 months
    c. Is adopted and does not know where her birth parents are
    d. Has a court order stipulating she is independent of her parents
    e. Is in the U.S. Army

22. Which of the following data should be included in an incident report regarding each incident?
    a. A patient was found on the floor in the bathroom. Include what you believe happened to result in the patient being on the floor.
    b. You administered an incorrect medication to a patient. Include the name, dose, and route of the medication administered.
    c. A patient fell while you were ambulating the patient in the hallway. Include vital signs assessed after the fall.
    d. A patient suffered a skin tear while you were assisting the patient to get out of bed. Include the location, size, and description of the skin tear.

Part 4. Application and Critical Thinking Questions

▶ *Scenario: Questions 23 through 25 refer to this scenario.*

You are caring for an 82-year-old female patient just admitted for a fractured tibia and fibula. While assessing the patient, you note multiple bruises over the patient's back and both upper arms. The patient is oriented to person but disoriented to place and time. The patient has no teeth or dentures. The patient's height is 5'6" and weight is 106 pounds. It is time for the evening meal and you bring the patient an edentulous diet ordered by the physician. The patient gulps the food down in only a couple minutes and asks for more, which you provide. While the patient is eating, the patient's daughter enters the room and begins to interact with the patient. During their conversation, you observe the patient flinching each time the daughter raises her hand to make a gesture. The daughter demonstrates a lack of patience and says several times to the patient, "Now, you have had enough to eat. You can't still be hungry."

23. What factors in the data presented contribute to your increasing concern for this patient's safety?

_____

_____

_____

_____

24. What further questions might you ask the patient later when you are alone with her?

_____

_____

_____

_____

25. What would be your legal responsibility regarding this information?

_____

_____

_____

_____

▶ *Scenario: Questions 26 through 29 refer to this scenario.*

Your patient is a 27-year-old woman who is scheduled for exploratory abdominal surgery in 2 hours. The physician has told you that he anticipates that he will find it necessary to perform a total hysterectomy during the exploratory abdominal surgery. You are performing preoperative patient teaching regarding this surgery and what the patient may expect before, during, and after the surgical procedure. The surgical consent form has been signed and is in the patient's chart. While teaching the patient, she comments, "I'll be so glad to get this surgery over with. I'm anxious to get rid of the pain. I'm so glad that this surgery will finally fix my stomach, you know? My husband and I were ready to start our family when I got sick and we want to get pregnant as soon as possible after I am well. We'd like to have three or four children eventually."

26. What about the patient's comments concerns you?

_____

_____

_____

_____

27. Do you feel comfortable sending the patient to surgery? Explain your answer.

_____

_____

_____

_____

28. What two actions should you take immediately?

_____

_____

_____

_____

29. If the surgery is performed without taking any further action, including the two actions in question 28, under which tort law could this situation fall?

_____

_____

_____

_____

Documentation Exercise

30. Following is a list of data. Some information is appropriate to include in an incident report and some is inappropriate. Think of an accident that might happen to a hospitalized patient. Complete the incident form at the end of this section (Fig. 3-1) for this faux accident, including only appropriate types of data.

Date and time the incident report is completed

Date and time of the incident

Names of all witnesses

Patient name

What the witnesses stated had happened

To the best of your ability, tell what you think what must have happened in your absence

Patient's age, sex, and diagnosis

Assessment of the patient's fall risk pre-incident

Where you were and what you were doing in another location when the incident occurred

What the witnesses assumed was the cause of the incident

Current vital signs

What the patient stated had happened

Assessment findings

Your age and sex

Name of the patient's physician

Time of notification of the physician

The physician's statement of the damage that could occur as a result of the incident

Treatment provided to the patient pre-incident

Treatment provided to the patient post-incident

Objective description of the patient's condition post-incident

				Report #_____	
				Date Received:_____	
				Initials:_____	

Kingfisher Regional Hospital
Unusual Occurrence Report

Date of Event:_____ Time of Event:_____ Department:_____

Patient Last Name:		First Name:		MI	
Patient #		Attending Physician:			
Visitor Last Name:		First Name		Phone:	
Employee Name:		Dept:			
Physician Name:		Specialty:			

Occurrence Category: (Circle most appropriate)

Fall	Treatment/Procedure	Equipment/Supplies	AMA	Diet Related
HIPAA Compliance	Medication Related	Narcotic Related	Delay in Treatment	Security
Loss of Personal Property	Patient Injury	Order Not Executed	Peer Review Related	Agency Nurse Related
Employee Injury	Visitor Injury	Restraint Related	Other:	

Provide a Brief Description of the Event:

\
\
\
\
\
\
\
\
\
\
\
\

What are the Contributing Factors? (Circle all that apply)

Individual:	System:
Knowledge, Skills, Experience: Unclear or Incomplete	Policies/Procedures Not In Place: Unclear, Outdated
Standard of Care or Practice: Non-Adherence to	Environmental: Staffing, Patient Acuity, Congestion
Documentation: Incomplete or Not Adequate	Communications and Work Flow: Intra & Inter Departmental
	Equipment Failure

Other: (Please Explain)

\
\
\

Submitted by:	Dept.	Date:

Figure 3.1 Incident report form. *(Courtesy of Kingfisher Hospital)*

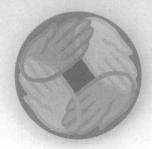

The Nursing Process and Decision Making

Name:
Date:
Course:
Instructor:

Part 1. Key Terms Review

Match the following Key Term(s) or italicized words from your text with the correct description.

_____ 1. Objective data

_____ 2. Primary data

_____ 3. Secondary data

_____ 4. Subjective data

a. Symptoms knowable only by the patient

b. Data obtained from a source other than the patient

c. Data that can be assessed through the senses

d. Data provided by the patient

Fill in the blank with the correct Key Term(s) or italicized words from your text.

5. A documented strategy that includes physician's orders, nursing diagnoses, and nursing orders is called the _____.

6. _____ is using competent reasoning and logical thought processes to determine the merits of a belief or action.

7. To avoid making decisions based on assumptions, nurses _____ the information they obtain.

8. The _____ is an overlapping, five-step method for decision making.

9. Creating a relationship of mutual trust is called establishing a _____.

10. The concise statement of a problem that the patient is experiencing as a result of his or her medical diagnoses is called the _____.

11. The signs and symptoms experienced by the patient that directly influence the nursing diagnosis are called the _____.

12. The _____ is the overall direction that will indicate improvement in a problem.

13. _____ are statements of measurable action for the patient within a specific time frame in response to nursing interventions.

14. When an individual nurse performs hands-on or one-on-one nursing interventions, it is called _____.

15. Activities that a nurse performs that do not involve hands-on or one-on-one patient care but nonetheless have an impact on the patient are called

    _____.

16. Actions the nurse performs that do not require a written order are called _____.

17. Actions the nurse performs that require a written order are called _____.

18. Nursing actions that involve working with other disciplines such as physical therapy or social services are called _____.

Part 2. Connection Questions

Choose the correct answer(s). In some questions, more than one answer is correct. Select all that apply.

19. Assume you are scheduled for clinical tomorrow. How would you obtain information about your patient so that you can begin to develop a plan of care?
    a. Read the nursing admission assessment and recent nurse's notes.
    b. Read the physician admission note and recent progress notes.
    c. Listen to the end-of-shift report at the nurse's station.
    d. Review the medication administration record and any treatment plans or notes.

20. Refer to the Real-World Connection feature called Critical Thinking in Patient Care located in Chapter 4 in your textbook. What did the nurse and the therapist do that is a characteristic feature of critical thinking?
    a. They made important observations.
    b. They made a difference in patient care.
    c. They thought they could get to the bottom of the problem.
    d. They made a conscious decision to think in a new way about the problem.

21. You are accepting a patient who is being transferred to your general care unit after 3 days in the intensive care unit (ICU) following a stroke. Many of the stroke symptoms have resolved and the patient needs only minimal physical and occupational therapy. Because the care is uncomplicated and you are busy with patients who are sicker, you ask the unlicensed assistant to develop the care plan, after which you will assess it and revise it as needed. Which of the following statements about your actions is true?
    a. This is fine; you may delegate care planning as long as a licensed nurse reviews it.
    b. This is fine as long as you choose the nursing diagnoses.
    c. This is not allowed because nursing decisions and care planning cannot be delegated.
    d. This is not allowed because the patient is coming from an ICU.

22. Your patient was admitted to the hospital with severe abdominal pain. It was determined that he had pancreatitis as a result of severely elevated triglycerides. He was also diagnosed with type 2 diabetes, and you plan to teach him about his diagnosis. He is not allowed anything by mouth yet because of the pancreatitis, is receiving IV fluids, and requires pain medication every 3 to 4 hours. You enter the room and let him know you want to discuss his health conditions with him. He responds by saying, "Not now, please, I just got my pain shot." Which of the following explains how the patient's comment reflects Maslow's hierarchy of needs?
    a. He has to have his safety and security needs met before he can address cognitive needs.
    b. Cognitive needs are less important than physical needs.
    c. He cannot deal with learning new issues while he feels physically uncomfortable.
    d. His discomfort is preventing him from cooperating.

Part 3. Review Questions

Choose the correct answer(s). In some questions, more than one answer is correct. Select all that apply.

23. A student in your class is given the name of a patient for whom she will provide care the following day in clinical. She goes to the unit, which specializes in diabetes care, to find out information and sees the patient sitting in a wheelchair with his chart in his lap. He is on his way to radiology for an x-ray. She notes that his left leg is amputated just below the knee and that his right foot is bandaged. Your class has been studying diabetes and the student knows that vascular problems and amputations are unfortunate complications of diabetes. She plans to study about diabetic foot care tonight so that she will be prepared for clinical the next day. Which of the following represents an accurate statement about her decision to study diabetic foot care?
    a. It reflects careful observation and good planning.
    b. The amputation and bandage are pretty obvious, so her plan is just common sense.
    c. She should read the patient's specific foot care program before reading about general diabetic foot care.
    d. She has made a serious thinking error.

24. Which step of the nursing process is concerned with identifying physical findings?
    a. Assessment
    b. Diagnosis
    c. Planning
    d. Implementation
    e. Evaluation

25. In which step of the nursing process would you look at outcomes?
    a. Assessment
    b. Diagnosis
    c. Planning
    d. Implementation
    e. Evaluation

26. In which step of the nursing process are priorities set?
    a. Assessment
    b. Diagnosis
    c. Planning
    d. Implementation
    e. Evaluation

27. In which step of the nursing process do you label problems?
    a. Assessment
    b. Diagnosis
    c. Planning
    d. Implementation
    e. Evaluation

28. Which step of the nursing process is most associated with action?
    a. Assessment
    b. Diagnosis
    c. Planning
    d. Implementation
    e. Evaluation

29. You enter the room to find your patient ashen and gasping for breath. Which part of the nursing process should you perform, formally or informally, in the first 5 minutes?
    a. Assessment
    b. Diagnosis
    c. Planning
    d. Implementation
    e. Evaluation
    f. All of the above

30. You are caring for a male patient who had a total hip replacement 3 days earlier. You have not cared for the patient before and are assessing him to establish a baseline of information about his health status. The patient states he felt feverish during the night and broke into a sweat. You check his temperature readings from the previous night and see that it was 99.2°F at midnight and 98.2°F at 6 a.m. It now is 99°F. Which of the following actions represents the best response to his statement and gives the best explanation for the action as it relates to critical thinking?
    a. Tell him not to worry because his temperature was only 99.2°F. This action shows that you understand normal trends in postoperative care and are applying them to unique situations.
    b. Make a mental note to check his temperature a few more times this shift. This action shows that you understand that assessment is the first and most important step in the nursing process.
    c. Assess him for signs and symptoms of an infection. This action shows that you are looking for data to validate the patient's comment.
    d. Tell him that a low-grade fever is normal after surgery. This shows that you are aware of common clinical conditions.

31. You have passed your NCLEX-PN examination and have just been employed as an LPN on a medical surgical unit. The registered nurse (RN) in charge asks you to do the admission assessment on a new patient who has just arrived by ambulance from a long-term care facility. The patient had undergone a total hip replacement within the previous 2 weeks and has developed a fever. You tell the nurse you thought an LPN could not do the admission assessment or, at most, could do only certain portions of it. The nurse, who is very busy, says, "Please just do it. I'll cosign it, so it will be fine." Which of the following actions should you take next?
    a. Call the supervisor to discuss the nurse's instructions to you.
    b. Refuse to do the admission assessment but offer to get the patient settled in, take his vital signs, and review the chart for orders.
    c. Check the facility's policy manual.
    d. Do the assessment as requested.

32. You are performing the daily assessment of your patient's status. You notice some purplish marks on her arm where the bandage for her IV had been and the skin is torn. Which of the following techniques did you use to obtain these data?
    a. Inspection
    b. Palpation
    c. Auscultation
    d. Percussion

33. To assess bowel sounds, which assessment technique will you use?
    a. Inspection
    b. Palpation
    c. Auscultation
    d. Percussion

34. Your patient has severe peripheral vascular disease (poor circulation) in both lower extremities. You document that the patient's pedal pulses are absent. Which assessment technique did you use to obtain these data?
    a. Inspection
    b. Palpation
    c. Auscultation
    d. Percussion

35. You are assisting the nurse practitioner (NP) with her assessment of an elderly, confused woman. You watch as the NP places her hand on the woman's back and then taps her own middle finger with her other hand. This assessment technique is called
    a. inspection.
    b. palpation.
    c. auscultation.
    d. percussion.

36. How is Maslow's hierarchy of human needs used by nurses in a clinical setting?
    a. It serves as a reminder of human growth and development across the life span.
    b. It is a framework for thinking critically.
    c. It helps in prioritizing nursing diagnoses and care.
    d. It outlines the basic psychological needs that people have when they are hospitalized and feeling vulnerable.

Indicate whether the following statements are True (T) or False (F).

_____ 37. The NANDA-I list of nursing diagnoses is the only source of nursing diagnoses available.

_____ 38. Nursing diagnoses and medical diagnoses both use the names of diseases.

_____ 39. By using a problem statement, the cause of the problem, and the defining characteristics of the problem, nursing diagnoses help identify interventions to address the problem.

_____ 40. Nursing diagnoses all contain the modifier "risk for."

_____ 41. A nursing diagnosis may be a one-part, two-part, or three-part statement.

_____ 42. Improvement in a patient's health problem is measured by how much progress the patient makes toward the goal, which is set by the nurse.

_____ 43. When a patient achieves the expected outcome, the nursing diagnosis is resolved.

_____ 44. The evaluation step of the nursing process is the step in which the plan of care is either changed or continued.

_____ 45. Implementation means putting the plan into action and performing the interventions.

_____ 46. LPNs/LVNs do not have a role in determining nursing diagnoses for the care plan.

_____ 47. Specified diagnoses are those that clearly apply to one defined patient need, so that any more description would only be redundant.

_____ 48. Wellness diagnoses are characterized by the phrase "ready for enhanced."

Choose the correct answer(s). More than one answer may be correct. Select all that apply.

49. Although nursing interventions vary widely, the initial steps you will take before performing an intervention are somewhat standard. Which of the following should be done before any nursing intervention?
    a. Determine if the patient's condition has changed in such a way that the order might no longer be appropriate.
    b. Gather needed equipment and supplies.
    c. Explain the procedure to the patient.
    d. Identify the patient using two methods of identification according to facility policy.
    e. Provide privacy.
    f. Wash your hands.

Part 4. Application and Critical Thinking Questions

Write a brief answer to the following questions.

50. Provide a rationale for why each step of the nursing process is important. Although it may seem that the importance of the steps is obvious, write at least one sentence for each step detailing how the step helps in making decisions about patient care.

_____

_____

_____

_____

_____

_____

51. You are caring for a child with pneumonia. An RN is developing the care plan and asks for your input. Discuss three ways you can contribute to the care plan.

_____

_____

_____

_____

_____

_____

52. It is important to remember that the nursing process is not static but dynamic. In other words, you do not perform a single step at a time beginning with assessment and ending with evaluation. Use the following scenario to discuss the dynamic nature of the nursing process: You enter a patient's room to find the patient ashen, short of breath, and complaining of chest pain. Your first actions include checking vital signs, measuring pulse oximetry, giving nitroglycerin, applying oxygen, and notifying the physician. Explain which steps of the nursing process you are performing.

_____

_____

_____

_____

_____

53. Using a physical problem you understand well (e.g., common cold, flu, or broken bone), list the common signs and symptoms, and identify whether they represent subjective or objective data. List any further explanation on the blank lines.

Subjective Data	Objective Data

_____

_____

_____

_____

_____

54. Take the following nursing diagnoses and prioritize them according to Maslow's hierarchy of human needs, and group them using the hierarchy terms: ineffective airway clearance, spiritual distress, decreased cardiac output, readiness for enhanced power, ineffective breathing pattern, risk for injury, chronic low self-esteem, risk for loneliness, and readiness for enhanced spiritual well-being.

_____

_____

_____

_____

_____

_____

_____   _____

_____   _____

_____   _____

Documentation Exercise

55. Using the steps for concept mapping of a care plan located near the end of Chapter 4
    in your textbook, map out a care plan for a patient with a common cold. Be creative
    with interventions.

Name: _____

Date: _____

Assessment + Data Collection

Nursing Diagnosis: _____

Outcome: _____

Intervention	Evaluation

Figure 4.1 Care plan.

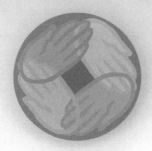

Documentation

Name:	_____
Date:	_____
Course:	_____
Instructor:	_____

Part 1. Key Terms Review

Fill in the blank with the correct Key Term(s) or italicized words from your text.

1. _____ is a style of charting that is much shorter and documents less data than some other charting styles and includes a list of nursing diagnoses identified from collected data, the actions you perform to address these nursing diagnoses, and evaluation of the effectiveness of those actions.

2. The type of charting that provides a continual chronological description of the patient's condition, complaints, problems, assessment findings of all systems, activities, treatments, nursing care provided, and the evaluations of effectiveness for each nursing intervention is known as _____.

3. The method of charting that provides the best organization of entries includes information verbalized by the patient and discerned with your senses, the problems you identify, the plan for what you are going to do to resolve the patient problems, the actual performance of those actions, measurement of their effectiveness, and whether or not you plan to revise the care plan is called

   _____.

4. A slightly more formal term that refers to the recording of data in a patient's chart and is synonymous with charting is _____.

5. A charting format in which the activities of daily living, vital signs, and assessment findings are charted on checklist-type flow sheets rather than writing them out as individual entries and only variances from "normal" are written as individual entries is known as _____

   _____.

6. _____ is a style of charting that includes objective and subjective assessment findings, the interventions you perform for the patient's problems, and how effective those interventions were. This style of charting does not use a compiled list of the patient's problems.

7. A type of flip chart with a page for each patient on the unit that contains a summary of care required by the patient and requires continual updating and maintenance by nursing staff is known as a _____.

Part 2. Connection Questions

Choose the correct answer(s). In some questions, more than one answer is correct. Select all that apply.

8. Which of the following is (are) a purpose of documentation?
   a. To provide a record for administration to prove that the nurses have earned their pay
   b. To provide a permanent record of medical diagnoses, nursing diagnoses, plan of care, care provided, and the patient's response to that care
   c. To serve as a punitive measure for nurses who will not do all the interventions
   d. To serve as a record of accountability for quality assurance, accreditation, and reimbursement purposes

9. The process of providing effective patient care that is delivered and evaluated continuously, systematically, and smoothly from one hour to the next, including through the staffing changes between shifts, is known as what?
   a. Internal assessment
   b. Accreditation
   c. Quality assurance
   d. Continuity of care

10. Which of the following statements is (are) true in reference to The Joint Commission?
   a. The Joint Commission audits medical records to verify facility compliance in meeting established health-care standards.
   b. The Joint Commission sets the standards by which the quality of health care is measured nationally and internationally.
   c. The Joint Commission seeks to improve safety and quality of care that health-care organizations provide to the public.
   d. The Joint Commission is a group of commissioned individuals who collectively represent all the medical insurance companies who set the standards for medical care reimbursement.

11. Why do insurance companies review medical records?
   a. Reimbursement is dependent on documentation of specific data in the medical record.
   b. Insurance reimbursement depends on the specific consents that the patient or family members have signed.
   c. Records help insurance companies to detect problems, less-than-desirable outcomes, or areas of weakness in the delivery systems so that improvements can be made.
   d. Because the medical record is the property of the patient's insurance company.

12. Which of the following statement(s) regarding a patient's hospital medical record is (are) accurate?
   a. All the information within the chart belongs to the patient.
   b. Access to a patient's medical record is restricted to the physician, the nurse, and the patient.
   c. HIPAA guarantees the patient the right to view his or her own medical record.
   d. The patient may not take the original medical record because it is the property of the hospital.
   e. The medical record belongs to the admitting physician.
   f. The hospital must provide the patient with a written explanation of how the patient's health information will be used.
   g. The patient has the right to a copy of any or all of his or her own medical records.

13. What happens to the Kardex page after a patient is discharged?
   a. It is disposed of in the trash.
   b. It remains with the chart because it is a part of the medical record.
   c. It is given to the patient for a record of his or her care.
   d. It is shredded or filed with the chart, dependent on facility policy.

14. What is the military time for 1:15 a.m.?
    a. 0115
    b. 1315
    c. 1115
    d. 1150

15. What time would the military time 2210 be?
    a. 10:22 a.m.
    b. 10:22 p.m.
    c. 2:21 a.m.
    d. 10:10 p.m.

16. Which of the following would be subjective data?
    a. Pain
    b. Itching
    c. Grimacing
    d. Flushing
    e. 124/74
    f. WBC-13,200
    g. Sleeping
    h. Snoring

17. Which of the following are sections of a source-oriented chart?
    a. Database
    b. Graphic sheet
    c. Laboratory
    d. Medication Administration Record
    e. Nurse's notes
    f. Physician's progress notes

18. Which of the following types of data should be included in weekly summaries in a long-term care facility?
    a. Use of prosthesis
    b. Activity level
    c. Length of time the resident has been at the facility
    d. Whether continent or incontinent of bowel and bladder
    e. Whether the resident can speak
    f. Whether the resident routinely has relatives and visitors
    g. Social activities in which the resident participates
    h. Staff members with whom the resident does not get along
    i. Ability to bathe and feed self, including type of bath
    j. Type of diet, percentage generally consumed
    k. Whether the resident is self-pay or third-party reimbursement

19. Which of the following charting "omissions" (meaning they were not charted) would carry additional risks just by the nature of the omission?
    a. The time a patient consumed his or her evening meal
    b. A rash and swelling noted during assessment
    c. The fact that the patient has a history of hemophilia
    d. A physician's order for a medication
    e. The nurse instructed the patient that he needs to increase oral intake
    f. Noting of a physician's order to make a patient NPO

20. You can safely delegate documentation of certain data to an unlicensed staff member. Which of the following data cannot be delegated?
    a. Administration of medication
    b. Graphing vital signs
    c. Items on a patient care flow sheet, such as type of bath, ambulation, or percentage of diet consumed
    d. Items on a patient care flow sheet, such as prn use of oxygen, that heart sounds are distinct, or presence of edema

Part 3. Review Questions

Indicate whether the following statements are True (T) or False (F).

_____21. Statistics such as rates of hospital-acquired infections, mortality rates, success rates of specific procedures, and number of incidents and accidents serve as factors of a medical facility's reputation.

_____22. Failure to document administration of a medication does not carry an increased risk.

_____23. A federal law known as OBRA mandates that an extensive assessment form called the MDS must be completed on every patient admitted to the hospital.

_____24. The omission of a patient's latex allergy in his medical history carries an increased risk.

_____25. An advantage of computerized documentation is that it is easy to read.

_____26. The primary disadvantage of charting by exception is the absence of specific data that might be useful in defense of your actions in a court of law.

_____27. When documenting patient teaching, the only thing that must be included is the subject that was taught and the methods used to teach the subject.

_____28. If your cursive writing is not legible, you must print your documentation.

_____29. The only time that it is okay to share your computer password with another student or coworker is if he or she is going to document vital signs for you.

Write a brief answer to the following questions.

30. What can you do to help ensure the intended recipient is the only one who receives a faxed medical record you send?

_____

_____

31. What do the letters S, O, A, P, I, E, R stand for in SOAPIER charting?

_____

_____

_____

_____

_____

_____

32. What do the letters P, I, E stand for in PIE charting?

_____

_____

_____

33. What do the letters D, A, R stand for in focus charting?

_____

_____

_____

_____

34. List at least 9 of the 10 categories of specific data that should be documented for every patient.

_____

_____

_____

_____

_____

_____

_____

_____

Choose the correct answer(s). In some questions, more than one answer may be correct. Select all that apply.

35. Which of the following rule(s) do(es) not apply to documentation?
    a. Avoid leaving blank lines.
    b. Write in complete sentences using correct grammar.
    c. Capitalize the first letter of the first word of each phrase.
    d. The only subjective data that you should document are that which the patient or patient's family members may tell you verbally.
    e. Use only approved abbreviations.
    f. Attempt to accurately label the patient's behaviors with terms that are descriptive.
    g. End each phrase or sentence with a period.

36. Guidelines for documentation include which of the following?
    a. All documentation for your shift must be signed after you have charted your last entry for the shift.
    b. All documentation must be done in cursive writing.
    c. Charting should be done in blocks of time to reduce the number of unnecessary entries.
    d. The date and time should be included with each entry.

37. The correct signature for documentation includes which of the following?
    a. First and last names
    b. First name, last initial, and credentials
    c. First initial, middle initial, last initial, and credentials
    d. First name, middle name, last name
    e. First initial, last name, and credentials

38. When used for documentation, which color ink will copy best?
    a. Black
    b. Red
    c. Green
    d. Purple

39. Occurrences that should be documented on an incident or variance report form include some of the following. Which ones are included?
    a. A patient fall
    b. A medication error
    c. A ¼-inch scrape on a visitor's leg from brushing the leg against the edge of the wheelchair
    d. A lack of supplies needed to perform a procedure
    e. A nursing assistant bumped her head on the television mounted on the wall
    f. An unsafe staffing situation for the number and type of patients on the unit

Part 4. Application and Critical Thinking Questions

Choose the correct answer(s). In some questions, more than one answer is correct. Select all that apply.

40. Some of the following documentation phrases include subjective terminology that needs to be changed to objective terminology. Select the phrases with subjective terms and underline the subjective word(s) that need(s) to be changed to objective.
    a. Snored loudly most of night between 0030 and 0530.
    b. Green purulent drainage increased from yesterday. ABD pad has 6" circle of drainage.
    c. Procedure tolerated well.
    d. ADA diet—ate 75% tolerated poorly.
    e. Bouncing foot almost continually. Rubbing hands and flicking finger with thumb at intervals. Verbally denies feeling nervous or anxious.
    f. Got mad while ambulating in the hall.
    g. Has a bad attitude.

41. Which of the following entries are succinct?
    a. I took her temp and it was up to 104.2 degrees Fahrenheit.
    b. After giving a complete bed bath, oral care was performed with toothpaste, toothbrush, and mouthwash. Lotion was applied liberally over arms, back, legs, feet, and hands. Her feet and back were massaged for quite a while.
    c. 18 Fr. Foley cath inserted without difficulty& hung to gravity drainage. Returned 275 mL clear pale yellow urine.
    d. The patient said she is really nauseated badly, but that she hasn't vomited yet. She asked for her nausea medication that comes in an injection.
    e. C/O constant sharp, stabbing pain in Rt. great toe, began 1 hr ago, now a 7 on 0–10 scale.

Situation Questions

For questions 42 through 44, first, underline the pieces of data in the scenario that are pertinent and should be documented. Second, make a charting entry: Write the data in succinct, accurate, and objective phrases that would be appropriate for documentation using the narrative charting format.

42. Scenario: You are working 7 a.m.–7 p.m. and it is 0830. Millie Norris has insulin-dependent diabetes and is hospitalized because her blood sugar has been out of control. She is acting differently than she did yesterday; she is awake but confused, her skin is flushed, hot, and dry. She slept normally on the previous shift, according to the report. You perform an FSBS and find that it is 475 mg/dL. You find Regular Insulin 8 units charted on the MAR for the previous evening at 2115.

_____

_____

_____

_____

_____

_____

43. Scenario: You are working the 7 p.m.–7 a.m. shift. It is now 2010. The patient is Mike Gibson, who has been admitted with pneumonia. In the report you were told that an antitussive (cough syrup) was administered to Mr. Gibson for frequent, nonproductive coughing at 1445 and acetaminophen for a headache at 1855. During your initial shift assessment he tells you that his headache is completely gone, but that he is feeling slightly short of breath and cannot stop coughing. You empty and clean his emesis basin, which contains a large amount of thick yellowish sputum, which he tells you just started to "come up" in the last hour or so. You find that he took his evening shower right after taking the acetaminophen. He tells you that it was a hotter-than-usual shower and it felt so good that he stayed in the shower for 20 to 25 minutes, when normally he jumps in, showers quickly, and gets out, staying 7 to 8 minutes at the most.

_____

_____

_____

_____

_____

_____

_____

_____

_____

44. Scenario: The patient is Marvin Bishop, who was admitted on 11/28/17 for abdominal pain to rule out appendicitis. You are working 7 a.m.–7 p.m. It is now 1305 and Mr. Bishop rings to tell you that he is nauseated, a new development, and that his right lower quadrant (RLQ) pain just escalated suddenly to a 10. He tells you that he must have something for pain now. You assess his abdomen and find that it is flat and not distended; he guards when you palpate the RLQ and right upper quadrant (RUQ), and he flinches and moans when you palpate and then release hand pressure applied over the RLQ area where he states he hurts the most.

_____

_____

Documentation Exercises

For questions 45 through 49, use the abbreviations found in Box 5-1.

45. **Note the vital signs and weight in the bottom rows of the graphic sheet, in the "Frequent vs. Monitoring / Reason" area (Fig. 5-1).** Scenario vital signs: The following vital signs and weight were taken on January 23, 2017, at the specified times for the patient in Room 324, Winona Weaver.

0700: BP-148/84, T-99.2, P-83, R-19, weight 134 pounds
1100: BP-156/86, T-100.4, P-91, R-20
1515: BP-150/82, T-102.4, P-102, R-26
1600: BP-152/88, T-103.1, P-104, R-27
1700: BP-148/80, T-101.2, P-100, R-25
1820: BP-146/78, T-100.4, P-92, R-22
1900: BP-144/78, T-99.8, P-80, R-18
2300: BP-132/74, T-99.2, P-74, R-17

The following vital signs were taken on January 24, 2017.
0300: BP-132/76, T-98.8, P-71, R-16
0700: BP-134/72, T-99.1, P-70, R-18, weight 133 pounds
1100: BP-141/78, T-101.2, P-84, R-21

Box 5–1

Commonly Used Health-Care Abbreviations

Abbreviations	Meaning	Abbreviations	Meaning
a⁻	before	BSC	bedside commode
ac	before meals	c⁻	with
ADLs	activities of daily living	ca	cancer
ad lib	as patient desires	cal	calories
AKA	above the knee amputation	cath	catheter
amb	ambulate, ambulatory	CBC	complete blood count
amp	ampule	CCU	coronary care unit; critical care unit
amt	amount	chem.	chemistry
ASAP	as soon as possible	CHF	congestive heart failure
ax	axillary	cm	centimeter
BE	barium enema	c/o	complained of
bid	twice per day	CO₂	carbon dioxide
BKA	below knee amputation	CPR	cardiopulmonary resuscitation
BM	bowel movement	CVA	cerebrovascular accident; stroke
BMR	basal metabolic rate	D&C	dilatation and curettage
BP	blood pressure	DM	diabetes mellitus
bpm	beats per minute	dsg or drsg	dressing
BR	bedrest	Dx	diagnosis
BRP	bathroom privileges	ECG or EKG	electrocardiogram

Continued

Box 5–1

Commonly Used Health-Care Abbreviations—cont'd

Abbreviations	Meaning	Abbreviations	Meaning
EEG	electroencephalogram	NGT	nasogastric tube
EENT	eyes, ears, nose, throat	NKA	no known allergies
ER	emergency room	NKDA	no known drug allergies
ETOH	alcohol	noc	night
F	female or Fahrenheit	NPO	nothing by mouth
FBS	fasting blood sugar	N/V/D	nausea, vomiting, diarrhea
FSBS	finger-stick blood sugar	O	oral
ft	foot or feet	O_2	oxygen
Fr	French (diameter size measurement)	OB	obstetrics
fx	fracture	OOB	out of bed
g	gram	OR	operating room
GI	gastrointestinal	ortho	orthopedics
gr	grain	os	mouth or opening
gtt(s)	drop/drops	OT	occupational therapy
GU	genitourinary	OTC	over the counter
GYN	gynecology	oz	ounce
HA	headache	p⁻	after
Hct	hematocrit	pc	after meals
Hgb	hemoglobin	PCA	patient controlled analgesia
h/o	history of	PO	by mouth
hob	head of bed	prn	as needed
HOH	hard of hearing	PT	physical therapy
H&P	history and physical	q	every
hr	hour	qid	4 times per day
HS	hour of sleep	R	rectal
ht	height	Rt	right
HTN	hypertension	RLE	right lower extremity
hyper	above or high	RLL	right lower lobe
ICU	intensive care unit	RLQ	right lower quadrant
ID	intradermal	RML	right middle lobe
IM	intramuscular	R/O	rule out
Inj	injection	RUE	right upper extremity
I&O	intake and output	RUL	right upper lobe
IV	intravenous	RUQ	right upper quadrant
IVP	intravenous push	Rx	prescription
IVPB	intravenous piggy-back	s⁻	without
L	liter	SCD	sequential compression device
lb	pound	SOB	short of breath
liq	liquids	SSE	soap-suds enema
LLE	left lower extremity	stat	immediately
LLL	left lower lobe	STD	sexually transmitted disease
LLQ	left lower quadrant	TB	tuberculosis
LMP	last menstrual period	tid	three times per day
LUE	left upper extremity	TO	telephone order
LUL	left upper lobe	TPR	temperature, pulse, respirations
LUQ	left upper quadrant	Tx	treatment
LOC	level of consciousness	UA	urinalysis
med	medication	VO	verbal order
mg	milligram	VS	vital signs
mL	milliliter	WBC	white blood count
MN	midnight	w/c	wheelchair
NAS	no added salt	WNL	within normal limits
NG	nasogastric	wt	weight

46. On a nurse's note form (Fig. 5-2), use the focus charting style to document the following scenario. Be succinct, accurate, and include all data. Be certain to close with your signature and credentials as a student nurse. RN students will use SN, LPN students will use SPN, and LVN students will use SVN as credentials unless instructed otherwise by your nursing instructor.

Scenario: Mary Elliott is in Room 333 and her hospital ID is #021481. Her BD is 2/14/82 and she was admitted 6/21/17.

Today's date: June 23, 2017. At 0815 Ms. Elliott complains of shortness of breath that worsens every time she gets up to the bathroom or just turns over in bed. Her pulse is strong. She appears pale and is coughing frequently and coughs up lots of greenish yellow sputum. Her respirations are 33, regular, and of even depth. Her skin is warm. At this time her SpO_2 is ninety percent without supplemental oxygen. Her skin is dry. Her pulse is 92 and regular. You have physician's orders to apply supplemental oxygen at three liters a minute using a nasal cannula for the delivery device. You perform this intervention. You also have an order for Guaifenesin syrup with codeine 2 teaspoons to be given orally every 4 hours prn. You administer this cough medication as ordered because she has not had any in more than 6 hours. You also obtain a bedside commode for her to use. You instruct her to not get up alone, but to call for assistance until the dyspnea has improved. Approximately 10 minutes after you apply the O_2, her SpO_2 is ninety-six percent, her respirations are 29 regular and even, and her pulse is 87 strong and regular. She is not quite as pale as she was. Her mucous membranes are nice and pink. She tells you that her breathing is easier now.

47. Use a nurse's note form (Fig. 5-3) to document the data in the following scenario using the PIE charting style. Be succinct, accurate, and thorough.

Scenario: Your patient's name is Judith Wykel. Her BD is 6/21/80 and her hospital ID is #0621199. She is in Room 555 and was admitted on 6/21/17.

Today's date is June 23, 2017. Ms. Wykel just reported that she vomited a small amount of bile and is still nauseated. She asks if she can have some medication for the nausea. The nausea is problem #4A on the Judith's problem list. She has Phenergan fifty milligrams ordered intramuscularly as needed every 3 to 4 hours for nausea or vomiting. The patient had her last injection at 0930 in the right ventrogluteal site, so you give it in the left ventrogluteal site at 1430. She is still nauseated but not vomiting as you administer the medication. When you reassess her nausea and vomiting at 1500, she reports that the nausea is getting better and that she has had no further vomiting.

48. On a nurse's note form (Fig. 5-4), document using the SOAPIER charting style the following scenario. Include all data and be succinct.

Scenario: Your patient is Misti Heston, who was born June 4, 1961. Her hospital ID is #112484 and she is in Room 651. She was admitted on May 28, 2017. She had abdominal surgery earlier this afternoon.

Today's date is May 29, 2017. At 2100 Misti Heston calls for a nurse and reports an uncomfortable wetness running down her abdomen below her abdominal dressing. Upon assessing the situation, you see pink-tinged serous drainage soaked through on her dressing, about a 4-inch diameter spot. There is a slowly dripping trail of the same type drainage coming from underneath the bottom of the dressing. The physician's orders state that dressing may be changed prn. You proceed to change the dressing. While you are changing the dressing, you note that the incision edges are well approximated. There is a Penrose drain on the left upper quadrant of her abdomen; just a few 4 × 4 gauze pads are placed over the end of the Penrose drain and they are saturated. After removing those saturated 4 × 4s, you can see that there is a large amount of serous drainage coming from the open distal end of the Penrose, but there is no drainage from the drain's insertion site. There is no edema of the drain insertion site or along the incision. You cleanse the incision and drain the insertion site with sterile normal saline and 4 × 4s. You apply bulk sterile 4 × 4s over the Penrose drain after applying a split drain gauze pad around the drain at the insertion site. You cover the entire site with two ABD pads for further absorbency and to help secure all the 4 × 4s, taping it securely with 1"-wide silk tape. Ms. Heston reports that it feels much better now that it is dry. You revise the care plan to add more bulk 4 × 4s over the Penrose until drainage slows.

49. Using the template in Figure 5-5 of your textbook, create your own Pocket Brains with the appropriate blanks for the required data that you will need to document for this patient on your 8-hour shift. You may alter the format to your own design; just be certain to include all necessary components and make it as functional as you can.

Scenario: You are receiving a verbal shift report for one of your assigned patients. You are using your own self-prepared form on which to write the necessary data that you will need to provide continuity of care for this patient.

The patient is Julie James and she is in Room 417. Her diagnosis is COPD and she has no known drug allergies. She is 69 years old. Her physician is Dr. Taylor. She was admitted on 8/24/17. She needs a CXR and a UA done today. Her medications on your 0700 to 1530 shift are due at 0900, 1200, 1400, and 1500. She has an IV with a 22-gauge intracath in her left forearm. It is infusing at the prescribed rate of 30 milliliters per hour with an IV pump. There is a physician's order to convert the IV to a saline lock this morning. Then a soap-suds enema is ordered. She can be up in the room as she desires and has a BSC in the room. Her vital signs are ordered every 2 hours. They will be due again beginning at 0800. She is to be up in the chair for her meals. She has continuous oxygen ordered at 2 liters per minute, delivered by a nasal cannula. SpO_2 will also be assessed with her vitals every 2 hours. She is to have a low-sodium diet. She is able to shower with standby assistance and should have mouth care after each meal. The physician has ordered I/O to be monitored. She has not had a BM in 2 days.

GRAPHIC CHART

(PT STAMP)

Hour →		07	11	15	19	23	03	07	11	15	19	23	03	07	11	15	19	23	03	07	11	15	19	23	03

Date: (×4)

Temperature: 106°, 105°, 104°, 103°, 102°, 101°, 100°, 99°, 98.6°, 98.5°, 98°, 97°, 96°

Pulse: 150, 140, 130, 120, 110, 100, 90, 80, 70, 60

Respirations: 50, 40, 30, 20, 10

BP →

WT →

Frequent vs Monitoring			Reason			Frequent vs Monitoring			Reason		
Date	Time	Temp	Pulse	Resp	BP	Date	Time	Temp	Pulse	Resp	BP

Figure 5.1 Graphic sheet.

| Patient _____ |
| ID# _____ RM _____ |
| BD _____-_____-_____ |
| Admit _____-_____-_____ |
| Physician _____ |

Mission Regional Hospital

Date	Time	Nurse's Notes

Figure 5.2 Nurse's note.

		Mission Regional Hospital

Patient _____
ID# _____ RM _____
BD _____-_____-_____
Admit _____-_____-_____
Physician _____

Date	Time	Nurse's Notes

Figure 5.3 Nurse's note.

| Patient _____ |
| ID# _____ RM _____ |
| BD _____-_____-_____ |
| Admit _____-_____-_____ |
| Physician _____ |

Mission Regional Hospital

Date	Time	Nurse's Notes

Figure 5.4 Nurse's note.

Figure 5.5 Pocket brains.

UNIT
2

Communicating and Understanding

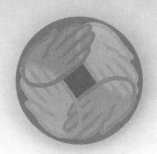

Communication and Relationships

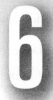
Name: _____	
Date: _____	
Course: _____	
Instructor: _____	

Part 1. Key Terms Review

Match the following Key Term(s) or italicized words from your text with the correct description.

_____ 1. Communication process

_____ 2. Feedback

_____ 3. Shared meaning

_____ 4. Verbal communication

_____ 5. Nonverbal communication

_____ 6. Body language

_____ 7. Congruent

_____ 8. Proxemics

a. To complete the communication process, a return message is sent by the receiver of the original communication to indicate the message has been received, processed, and comprehended

b. The conscious use of words, either spoken or written

c. The communication revealed through facial expressions, posture, body position, behavior, gestures, touch, and general appearance

d. Facial expressions, posture, body position, behavior, gestures, touch, and general appearance

e. The distance, or personal space, people place between themselves and others

f. An exchange of information, feelings, needs, and preferences between two people

g. Mutual understanding of the meaning of a message

h. Agreement between verbal and nonverbal communications

Fill in the blank with the correct Key Term(s) or italicized words from your text.

9. Using all the senses to interpret verbal and nonverbal messages is called _____.

10. _____ is patient centered and promotes a greater understanding of a patient's needs, concerns, and feelings.

11. Words can have two layers of meaning. _____ refers to the literal meaning, whereas _____ refers to the emotional associations attached to a word.

12. Two people are said to have a _____ when their relationship is characterized by mutual trust and understanding.

13. The ability to identify intellectually (not emotionally) with the experience, feelings, thoughts, or attitudes of others is called _____.

14. _____ is the inability to speak or understand language.

Part 2. Connection Questions

Choose the correct answer(s). In some questions, more than one answer is correct. Select all that apply.

15. Today is your first day on an Alzheimer's unit in a long-term care facility. Which of the following is the best way to begin to establish a connection with your patients?
    a. Have a peer formally introduce you to the patients.
    b. Smile at the patients.
    c. Sit among the patients.
    d. Read aloud to the patients.

16. Multiple areas of the brain are involved with all forms of communication. Which of the following is the likely outcome if your patient has a stroke that affects the left frontal lobe (Broca's area)?
    a. Loss of ability to perceive touch
    b. Loss of vision
    c. Loss of ability to formulate thoughts
    d. Loss of movement in muscles that control speech

17. Which communication form will be compromised if your patient has a stroke that affects the occipital lobe?
    a. Loss of ability to perceive touch
    b. Loss of vision
    c. Loss of ability to make gestures
    d. Loss of movement in muscles that control speech

18. Which communication form will be compromised if your patient has a stroke that affects the parietal lobes?
    a. Loss of ability to perceive touch
    b. Loss of vision
    c. Loss of ability to make gestures
    d. Loss of movement in muscles that control speech

19. When communicating with patients of various ages, it is important to match your communication strategies to the patients'
    a. Style of communication.
    b. Developmental stage.
    c. Reading level.
    d. Cultural sensitivity.

20. When communicating with older adults, it is important to be aware of
    a. Any impairments in vision or hearing.
    b. Chronic pain issues.
    c. Dementia that interferes with communication.
    d. Environmental distractions.

21. When caring for a patient in clinical, you are aware that he only responds with "yes" or "no" when you talk with him. What strategies could you use to better communicate with this patient?
    a. Rely on nonverbal communication only, watching him closely at all times.
    b. Try to find out his favorite sports team and talk with him about it.
    c. Use open-ended questions when eliciting information from him.
    d. Ask his family how to get him to talk more.

Part 3. Review Questions

Indicate whether the following statements are True (T) or False (F).

_____22. Communication between two people is called one-sided communication because one side gives communication and the other side receives the communication.

_____23. Communication is the process of informing.

_____24. Interpreting information is not a part of communication but is a part of listening.

_____25. People will let you know how well you are communicating by giving you feedback.

_____26. Shared meaning refers to two people deciding what another person meant.

Choose the correct answer(s). In some questions, more than one answer is correct. Select all that apply.

27. You enter your patient's room and find him sitting in a chair with his eyes closed. He has a grimace on his face and is holding his body rigidly. You ask him if he is feeling okay and he says, "Yes, I'm fine. Really." Which of the following best explains this situation in terms of communication?
    a. He is communicating to you that he's fine.
    b. His verbal and nonverbal messages are congruent.
    c. His verbal and nonverbal messages are incongruent.
    d. He is sarcastic, but it is understandable.

28. You are helping wash a 27-year-old female patient who has had back surgery. Of the following, which is the best way to communicate your respect for the fact that you are "invading" her personal space?
    a. Pull the curtains so no one can see you or the patient while you help with her bath.
    b. Pull the curtains, give her a dry towel, and tell her she can use it to "cover up."
    c. Pull the curtains and ask her how you can help her.
    d. Pull the curtains and tell her to wash her face and hands, then you will wash her back, and then she can "finish."

29. You ask an LPN on your team to interview a patient being admitted for surgery. You walk by the room and observe that the nurse is seated on the chair while the patient is seated on the bed. She is leaning forward slightly. By her body position you would conclude that:
    a. She is conducting the interview in an appropriate manner.
    b. She is too casual and should not be sitting.

30. Your patient has an infected wound with a lot of dead tissue called _eschar_ that is preventing healing. The doctor plans to debride the wound, which means to remove the dead tissue. You go in to prepare the patient for the procedure, which is done right at the bedside. Which of the following is the best way to communicate what will happen?
    a. "The doctor is going to cut away all the black, dead skin."
    b. "The doctor is going to debride the eschar."
    c. "The doctor is going to remove dead tissue so the wound can heal."
    d. "The doctor is going to clean the wound."

31. The language used during communication has a significant impact on how that communication is received. Which of the following statements can be used as a guide for communicating a plan of care to your teenage patient and her family?
    a. Speak to all of them as mature adults.
    b. Speak to the teenager in common, widely acceptable slang terms to put her at ease.
    c. Use the correct medical terminology when describing the plan to all of them.
    d. Use common, everyday language to describe the plan.

32. Acceptable, polite communication styles between professionals and their patients vary greatly among different cultures. Acceptable styles also vary within cultures. When approaching a patient from a cultural background other than your own, you should
    a. Maintain distance and avoid direct eye contact to be on the safe side.
    b. Observe how the family interacts and take your cues from that.
    c. Ask another professional from that cultural background for advice, if possible.
    d. Find out information about that culture from a different source, such as a pertinent Web site or text.

33. Nonverbal language can be expressive. As a nurse and a human being, you may experience negative feelings toward a patient, even though you try to overcome it, and you can strongly convey this negativity by your attitude. Which of the following is the best course of action for you should you find you have negative feelings toward a patient?
    a. Ask to be reassigned.
    b. Maintain a greater distance between you and the patient, which will provide a buffer for your feelings.
    c. Be aware of the attitude you display by exhibiting open, focused, nonverbal communication.
    d. Communicate your feelings to the patient in a nonjudgmental manner.

34. Active listening is
    a. Hearing what the patient has to say and then providing direction or advice.
    b. Hearing what the patient has to say and then expressing your feelings about the content.
    c. Hearing what the patient has to say, being attentive to nonverbal messages, and providing feedback.
    d. Hearing what the patient has to say, being attentive to nonverbal messages, and providing an interpretation to the patient.

Communication styles vary. Match the following statements to the communication styles described in the text. Assume you need to talk with an aide about a dressing change that has not been done.

_____35. "You need to understand that your work reflects on me."
     a. Assertive
     b. Avoidant
     c. Aggressive

_____36. "I want to talk with you about Mrs. G's dressing change. It was supposed to have been changed 2 hours ago."

_____37. "I'm going to change Mrs. G's dressing; I see you didn't get to it. Did you get busy?"

Write a brief answer to the following questions.

38. Using the DESC communication method as a guide, explain why describing the behavior is important as the first step.

    _____

    _____

    _____

    _____

    _____

39. In the DESC method, the E stands for "Explain." What needs to be explained and why?

    _____

    _____

    _____

    _____

40. Stating the desired outcome is the third step in the DESC communication method. Explain why you think this is important.

    _____

    _____

    _____

    _____

41. The C step of the DESC method is optional, depending on the circumstances. Explain what the C step is and why it may be needed.

    _____

    _____

    _____

    _____

Match the following therapeutic communication techniques to the correct definition.

_____42. Providing general leads

_____43. Using silence

_____44. Offering self

_____45. Open-ended questions or statements

_____46. Restatement

_____47. Seeking clarification

_____48. Reflection

_____49. Looking at alternatives

_____50. Giving information

_____51. Summarizing

a. Repeat same words back to the patient

b. Discourages answering questions with one or two words

c. Relate in different words the heart of what a patient said

d. Provide relevant data

e. Helps patients explore options when making decisions

f. Using pauses of up to several minutes without verbalizing

g. Restate the important points

h. Helps to verify that the message sent was what was intended

i. Encourages initiation or elaboration of a conversation

j. Shows concern and willingness to help

Choose the correct answer(s). In some questions, more than one answer is correct. Select all that apply.

52. Which of the following are barriers to communication?
    a. Using clichés
    b. Asking personal, probing questions
    c. Being frank about disapproval
    d. Standing over a seated person

53. A patient expresses fears about her upcoming surgery. The nurse responds, "You really don't have to worry. You have a great doctor and everything will turn out fine." Why is this statement a barrier to communication?
    a. It diminishes the patient's concerns.
    b. It is not a complete answer; the nurse should provide more information.
    c. It is equivalent to telling the patient to not talk about her fears.
    d. Providing reassurance is not therapeutic.

54. How can you communicate in an urgent situation?
    a. Use the SBAR communication format, which, if followed, will cover all aspects of communicating in a crisis.
    b. Use the SBAR format, allow your voice to reflect the urgency of the situation, and make sure your movements are purposeful and focused.
    c. Allow your voice to reflect the urgency of the situation, make sure your movements are purposeful and focused, and inform others of what you think is wrong.
    d. Allow your voice to reflect the urgency of the situation, make sure your movements are purposeful and focused, and let the most senior person in the room do the communicating.

55. A patient on your unit is very angry and hard to care for. She frequently belittles her caretakers. You have taken care of her for 2 days and ask the nurse manager to assign the patient to someone else. The nurse manager does as you ask, but the nurse she chooses comes to you and says, "This isn't fair at all! She is your patient and you are dumping her on me!" Which of the following alternatives is the best way to begin to resolve this conflict?
    a. Go back to the nurse manager and ask her to smooth things out.
    b. Tell the nurse privately that you needed an emotional break from the patient.
    c. Apologize to the nurse, take the patient back, and give the nurse one of the patients that had been assigned to you.
    d. Suggest that the nurse has not had the patient in a while and that it is her turn.

56. You work the day shift. A nurse on the evening shift, one whom you frequently report off to, is often 20 minutes late. She says it isn't her fault because she leaves in time for work, but the parking lot is so full when she arrives that she has to wait for a space to open up. Which of the following statements on your part reflects a good approach to resolving this conflict?
    a. "I have to be home on time for my kids. If you're late, I get nervous and worried."
    b. "You have to allow more time for parking. You make me late getting home for my kids and that is really wrong."
    c. "Think about how you would feel if the night shift was late most of the time."
    d. "I've put up with this for a long time now. I'm going to speak with the nurse manager about this."

57. Your patient had spine surgery 2 days ago and is scheduled for discharge tomorrow. He has been taking narcotic pain relievers every 4 hours around the clock. You note that the patient has not had a bowel movement since surgery. You know that the narcotics can be constipating and you think it would be best if the problem is handled prior to the patient leaving for home. There is no order on the chart for a laxative. From the following possible actions, choose which you think represents the most focused and necessary thing(s) for you to do as you prepare to call the doctor for a verbal order for a laxative.
    a. Gather information about the patient's usual bowel habits; ask if he feels constipated and if he has used laxatives in the past.
    b. Ask the patient what laxative has worked for him in the past.
    c. Ask the patient to try to have a bowel movement.
    d. Get the chart and have a pen ready.

Indicate whether the following statements are True (T) or False (F).

58. _____ Downward communication is communication with people you supervise.

59. _____ When you communicate effectively and professionally, you are role modeling, too.

60. _____ As a team leader, you have a responsibility to tell the people you supervise about your facility's policies and procedures.

61. _____ When assigning tasks to a team, you should explain how one task relates to another even if two different people are doing the tasks separately. This is called "job rationale."

62. _____ The shift-to-shift report is so important that The Joint Commission has made it a patient safety goal.

63. _____ It is not important for the shift report to be standardized in a facility, but it is important that the nurses coming on duty have plenty of time to ask questions.

64. _____ Giving reports to the oncoming shift is considered confidential.

65. _____ Select a sequence to present each patient's report so you will be less likely to forget something.

Choose the correct answer(s). In some questions, more than one answer is correct. Select all that apply.

66. The basis of the nurse–patient relationship is
    a. Admiration.
    b. Integrity.
    c. Trust.
    d. Caring.

67. You are interviewing a new patient who is being admitted to the psychiatric unit. Your technique in this interview will largely be
    a. Nondirective with many open-ended questions.
    b. Directive, with many closed-ended questions.
    c. Directive with many open-ended questions.
    d. Nondirective with many closed-ended questions.

68. Communicating with the hearing impaired can be a challenge. Which of the following techniques has been identified as helpful?
    a. Facing the person and getting his or her attention before starting to communicate
    b. Speaking clearly with markedly increased volume
    c. Speaking to the patient, not the interpreter, if there is one present
    d. Eliminating background noise or other distractions

Part 4. Application and Critical Thinking Questions

Write a brief answer to the following questions.

69. Explain how to enhance communication with a patient who is mechanically ventilated.

_____

_____

_____

_____

70. Describe how one can communicate with a patient who is comatose or unresponsive.

_____

_____

_____

_____

_____

_____

71. Discuss ways to improve upward communication in a facility.

_____

_____

_____

_____

_____

_____

72. The United States is becoming increasingly culturally diverse. Discuss two or three cultural factors that can interfere with nurse–patient communication and how you would overcome these obstacles.

_____

_____

_____

_____

_____

73. Develop a sequence for giving a report that will cover everything yet still be succinct. You can write this as a list or a series of steps. For example, you can write, "#1: Name, age, room number and doctor. #2: Diagnosis," and so on.

_____

_____

_____

_____

_____

Documentation Exercise

▶ *Scenario: Question 74 refers to this scenario.*

Your patient is a 14-year-old female, Charlene Jefferson, who has chronic renal failure from an inherited disorder. She has been started on dialysis and has a dialysis shunt in her left forearm. She is refusing to eat and will not speak to her doctors. Her doctors told her she will have to get a feeding tube if she does not eat. Based on your understanding of developmental issues, you believe Charlene is sad and angry about her diagnosis and probably does not like that she looks different because of the shunt in her arm. You realize that addressing all the issues will take several conversations, but your goal now is to establish a rapport with Charlene. You have just a few minutes and you enter her room. You introduce yourself and give her a big smile. You pull up a chair and sit with her so that you are at eye level with her. You have a relaxed posture but focus your attention on her by making eye contact.

"Hi, Charlene, my name is Cathy. I'm your nurse today. How are you doing?"

Charlene quietly says, "Okay," and stares out the window.

"I sense you're not happy, Charlene, what happened?" you ask.

Charlene tells you a little bit about her health issues and ends by saying, "I hate having this problem. I feel like a freak!"

"Do you feel different from your friends?" you ask. When she nods her head yes, you say, "I really want to help you, Charlene. Can we set up a time to talk later today?"

Charlene nods yes and you determine that you can come back at 11 a.m. to talk with her. You come back at 11 a.m. on the dot, sit down, and smile at her. You change your facial expression to one of concern, and say, "Let's pick up where we left off, Charlene. Tell me about your friends and how you feel different." Charlene begins to open up a bit about her life, expressing some general anger at her situation and her fears that she will get sicker.

You are aware that Charlene needs information and hope. You provide her with written handouts on renal failure and hemodialysis. She asks you about a kidney transplant. You explain a bit about how a transplant works and offer to have a member of the transplant team drop by and visit with her. Charlene says she is very interested in hearing more, so you tell her that you will arrange it.

74. Use the nurse's note (Fig. 6-1) at the end of the chapter to document your interaction with Charlene.

		Mission Regional Hospital
Patient _____		
ID# _____ RM _____		
BD _____-_____-_____		
Admit _____-_____-_____		
Physician _____		

Date	Time	Nurse's Notes

Figure 6.1 Nurse's note.

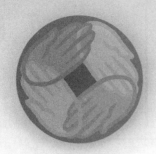

Promoting Health and Wellness

7

Name:	_____
Date:	_____
Course:	_____
Instructor:	_____

Part 1. Key Terms Review

Match the following Key Term(s) or italicized words from your text with the correct description.

_____ 1. Prodromal phase

_____ 2. Recovery phase

_____ 3. Symptomatic phase

_____ 4. Seeking help phase

_____ 5. Dependency phase

a. Patient agrees to advice and care by health-care providers

b. Patient contacts health-care provider

c. Disease-specific signs and symptoms resolve

d. Disease-specific signs and symptoms not yet present

e. Observable signs and symptoms present

Fill in the blank with the correct Key Term(s) or italicized words from your text.

6. _____ is a nonspecific response of the body to any demand made on it.

7. _____ is the ability to positively adjust to changes that occur in an individual's world.

8. A sympathetic nervous system reaction to perceived threats that results in the release of adrenaline, cortisol, and other hormones is called the _____.

9. Skills that all individuals use to manage everyday stress are called _____.

10. A scale that has a positive extreme at one end and the opposite extreme at the other end is called a

_____.

11. _____ is the ability of individuals to understand basic health information and to use that information to make good decisions about their health.

12. A condition or disorder lasting for 6 months or longer and is characterized by intensifying or improving symptoms is called a

_____.

13. A condition or disorder that strikes suddenly and lasts for a limited time is called an

    _____.

14. A report issued by the Department of Health and Human Services and called _____ highlights objectives related to disease prevention and health promotion for the American people.

15. Chronic illness is characterized by periods of either minimal symptoms or a complete absence of symptoms, called _____, and periods of worsening symptoms, called

    _____.

16. _____ are physiological, psychological, or genetic elements that contribute to the development of an illness or disease.

Part 2. Connection Questions

Write a brief answer to the following question.

17. Describe the "fight-or-flight response." List at least three physiological changes that occur and how these changes might help in a situation in which the individual must either fight back or flee.

    _____

    _____

    _____

    _____

    _____

    _____

Choose the correct answer(s). In some questions, more than one answer is correct. Select all that apply.

18. What is one of the main objectives of the body's fight-or-flight response?
    a. Keep electrolyte levels normal.
    b. Get more oxygen to certain organs and muscles.
    c. Raise the hemoglobin level.
    d. Keep the blood from clotting excessively.

19. What effects does the fight-or-flight response have on the cardiovascular system?
    a. Constricts blood vessels in the center of the body, dilates peripheral blood vessels, and increases heart rate
    b. Increases pumping of the heart, constricts peripheral blood vessels, and dilates central blood vessels
    c. Decreases cardiac output, raises blood pressure, and dilates blood vessels
    d. Increases heart rate, decreases respiratory rate, and constricts blood vessels

20. One action of the fight-or-flight response is to convert glycogen to glucose. What is the purpose of this action?
    a. To decrease appetite
    b. To increase respiratory rate
    c. To increase energy
    d. To decrease fluid loss

21. What happens to the nervous system once the threat is removed and the fight-or-flight response is no longer needed?
    a. Sympathetic nervous system reverses fight-or-flight response.
    b. Parasympathetic nervous system reverses fight-or-flight response.
    c. Central nervous system reverses fight-or-flight response.
    d. Peripheral nervous system reverses fight-or-flight response.

22. Your patient, Ms. Hernandez, has been admitted to the hospital with a bowel obstruction (blockage of the bowel, preventing bowel contents from advancing through the gastrointestinal tract). She has had a nasogastric tube for several days, but the obstruction has not resolved and she is scheduled for a large-bowel resection (surgical correction of the obstruction) the following day. You enter her room at 10 p.m. to check her IV and notice that she is crying. Which of the following represents the best action for you to take at this time?
    a. "I see you are crying. Do you want me to check if the doctor ordered something for you to calm your nerves?"
    b. "It's late and I'm sure you're tired and upset. I'll get you a shot to help you sleep."
    c. "Hello, Ms. Hernandez. Are you worried about your surgery? I'm sure I would be, too; but don't be. Your doctor is very good and everything will be fine. What can I do for you now?"
    d. "Hi, Ms. Hernandez, you seem upset. Can you tell me what's worrying you? Would you like me to explain more about the surgery?"

23. Which is an inappropriate intervention for the nurse to use for a patient who is experiencing increased stress due to hospitalization?
    a. Ask if the patient has any questions before performing a procedure or administering a medication.
    b. Pull up a chair and spend a few minutes listening to concerns the patient has about his or her diagnosis or care.
    c. Offer a back massage or warm drink if the patient is having difficulty sleeping.
    d. Explain that everyone who is in the hospital feels the same way and that things are never as bad as they seem when you are sick.

Part 3. Review Questions

Choose the correct answer(s). In some questions, more than one answer is correct. Select all that apply.

24. At any given time, most of us are neither completely healthy nor completely sick. We have the capacity to be healthier and the potential to become very sick. This concept is described as
    a. Healthy People 2020.
    b. The circle of life.
    c. The wellness–illness continuum.
    d. The health scale.

25. A definition of wellness or health would include
    a. Good physical condition only.
    b. Good physical health and the absence of mental illness.
    c. The absence of physical disease or mental disorders.
    d. Maximized physical and emotional health including the concept of well-controlled disease processes.

26. Dunn's theory of high-level wellness includes the concept of health or sickness as it relates to an individual's
    a. Environment.
    b. Financial status.
    c. Age.
    d. Medical history.

27. In Fitzpatrick's conceptualization of health, a person's health is viewed as
    a. A dynamic state that changes continuously through the lifetime.
    b. A static state influenced by financial status, environment, and health promotion activities.
    c. An emotional/physical state existing on a continuum of functional to dysfunctional.
    d. A changeable state influenced by self-care activities.

Write a brief answer to the following questions.

28. Choose two of the focus areas for Healthy People 2020 and discuss how you would help a patient to improve his or her health in relation to these two areas.

_____

_____

_____

_____

_____

_____

_____

_____

_____

_____

29. Discuss the consequences of a patient having poor health literacy.

_____

_____

_____

_____

Choose the correct answer(s). In some questions, more than one answer is correct. Select all that apply.

30. Which of the following are risk factors for illness?
    a. Genetic variation
    b. Psychological predisposition
    c. Environmental exposure
    d. Lifestyle choices

31. An important concept to understand about risk factors is that some are modifiable and some are not. Which of the following risk factors are modifiable?
    a. Tobacco use
    b. Family history of ovarian cancer
    c. Age
    d. Gender

Write a brief answer to the following question.

32. List three modifiable risk factors and correlate them to specific chronic illnesses.

_____

_____

_____

Indicate whether the following statements are True (T) or False (F).

33. _____ Stress results from a negative life event and it makes us more susceptible to illness.

34. _____ The elimination of stress as a risk factor for illness is possible through changes in lifestyle.

35. _____ Failure to adapt to stress can lead to death.

36. _____ The alarm phase of stress occurs when the body is first confronted with a threat.

37. _____ The body can resist stress indefinitely.

38. _____ When the body reaches the exhaustion stage of stress, the individual will get sick or die.

39. _____ Individuals adapt to stress by using coping strategies.

Choose the correct answer(s). In some questions, more than one answer is correct. Select all that apply.

40. Coping strategies may or may not be effective in managing stress. Which of the following variables will increase the effectiveness of an individual's coping strategies?
    a. Age of 65 years or older
    b. Well-controlled chronic illness
    c. Supportive family and friends
    d. Viewing the stressor as an enemy

41. Homeostasis refers to
    a. Static state of illness.
    b. Balance in the internal environment.
    c. Successful control of external environment.
    d. State of feeling well and happy.

42. Your friend is planning her marriage and is acting as a buffer between her mother and her future mother-in-law. She is excited about the wedding and honeymoon, and all the details are falling into place. She tells you she is so excited that her heart has been racing, which results in her feeling fearful and light-headed for a few minutes. Which of the following explanations best describes what your friend is experiencing?
    a. She is excited and probably somewhat tired out from all the planning.
    b. She may be drinking too much coffee.
    c. She is having panic attacks from too much stress.
    d. She is feeling normal effects for this stage in her life; in other words, a little light-headedness and fear are natural in this situation.

43. Which of the following actions will help combat stress?
    a. Getting 8 hours of sleep a night
    b. Learning deep breathing exercises
    c. Avoiding work you have to do
    d. Eating regular meals

44. Which of the following are overarching goals of Healthy People 2020?
    a. Attain high-quality, longer lives free of preventable disease, disability, injury, and premature death.
    b. Require all Americans under the age of 50 years to participate in an organized exercise program.
    c. Create social and physical environments that promote good health for all.
    d. Promote quality of life, healthy development, and healthy behaviors across all life stages.
    e. Limit sales of unhealthy beverages to 16 ounces or less per serving.

45. To determine a person's health literacy, the nurse asks the person to
    a. read aloud an information page about an ice-cream label.
    b. answer six questions about a specific ice-cream label.
    c. answer random questions after reading a short article about healthy behaviors.
    d. determine whether a serving of ice cream is or is not a healthy food choice by reading the label on the carton.

Part 4. Application and Critical Thinking Questions

Write a brief answer to the following question.

46. When a person is in a situation where his or her state of health is favorable, but the environment is not favorable, the person is in which of Dunn's quadrants?

_____

47. Review Table 7-2, Defense Mechanisms, in your textbook. Examine the information about denial, regression, and conversion reaction. Give an original example of the use of each one.

_____

_____

_____

_____

_____

_____

48. Apply your understanding of stressors, coping strategies, and defense mechanisms by identifying them in the following scenario. Write the name of the correct defense mechanism in the circle at the end of a sentence, if a defense mechanism is used. Or write the word(s) "stressor" or "coping strategies" in the circle, if it is an example of one of these. Two are filled in for you as examples.

Your patient, Mrs. Chan, is a 55-year-old female who has just been diagnosed with multiple sclerosis (stressor). Her symptoms currently are mild and the doctor cannot be sure if they will progress or at what rate they will progress. Mrs. Chan works with her husband in their business ( ). She has four children, three of whom have left the home and one who is still in college. Her husband's parents, whom Mrs. Chan does not like, live with them, and Mrs. Chan does all the housework and food preparation ( ). Mrs. Chan, immediately after hearing the diagnosis, thinks to herself that the doctors are probably wrong (denial). Subconsciously she is afraid she will not be able to work as hard as she normally does, which will make it harder for her husband. She is not conscious of these fears but decides to work even harder at home and in the business ( ). She blames the stress of having her in-laws living with her for getting this illness ( ) and wishes they would move away . She feels guilty for having these feelings, and when she is home she lavishes praise on her mother-in-law ( ). Mrs. Chan begins to realize that some days are worse than others and she attributes that to her husband's mood swings ( ). She decides to go back to yoga, which she did in the past and which she found relaxing. She also finds that she is more relaxed in the evenings if she drinks two or three glasses of wine ( ). Another way she feels more in control is by searching Internet sites to find more information about MS ( ). She feels better when she realizes that she is not as sick as many of the other people in chat rooms and support sites.

Documentation Exercise

▶ *Scenario: Question 49 refers to this scenario.*

It is 7/15/2017 at 8:15 a.m. and your 58-year-old patient, Mrs. Anita Lombardi, has an upper respiratory tract infection. Her date of birth is 5/20/1957, her hospital identification number is 111353, and she is in Room 133. She was diagnosed 1 year ago with chronic obstructive pulmonary disease (COPD). COPD is characterized by difficulty breathing resulting from damaged alveoli and other factors. It is associated with an abnormal amount of inflammation in the lungs and usually gets worse over time. Patients with COPD are susceptible to respiratory tract infections that can quickly cause difficulty with their breathing.

You note that Mrs. Lombardi has been hospitalized four times in the past year for respiratory infections. As you are taking her vital signs, you ask how she cares for herself at home. Mrs. Lombardi responds that she is very frustrated—she has been in the hospital "at least five times" this year, is constantly tired, and can no longer participate in activities she once enjoyed such as dancing. She works in a day-care center, and keeping up with the kids is getting hard for her. She says she feels like she is "drowning" half the time and has copious secretions that she coughs up several times a day. "It's embarrassing to be sick all the time," she says, and appears on the verge of tears. "It seems like I get sick so fast. One minute I'm okay and the next minute I'm in the emergency department feeling like I can't get my breath and am going to die. I can't live like this; can you do anything to help me?" she asks. You tell Mrs. Lombardi you will be back at 10 a.m. to teach her ways she can manage her condition better.

You return at 10 a.m. and begin teaching Mrs. Lombardi strategies to reduce her anxiety and manage her fears. You teach her about the importance of balancing activity with rest periods and what exercises she can do to improve her strength and stamina. Mrs. Lombardi says the exercises are easy enough for her to perform on a daily basis.

You return at 2 p.m. to complete her teaching because she will be discharged the next day. You and Mrs. Lombardi discuss ways to avoid infection including washing her hands frequently, which is especially important given that she works at a day-care center, avoiding contact with people with respiratory infections, and performing good oral hygiene. You teach her how to recognize signs and symptoms of infection and worsening respiratory status, and when to call her doctor before her condition gets serious. Finally, you recommend she get a pneumococcal vaccination and annual influenza vaccinations as preventive measures.

Mrs. Lombardi is able to repeat all the major points of the teaching plan. She has an appointment with her physician for the following week and will get her vaccinations then. She says she is grateful to have information she can use to help her take care of herself.

49. Please document this scenario in the nurse's notes (Fig. 7-1).

Patient _____ ID# _____ RM _____ BD _____-_____-_____ Admit _____-_____-_____ Physician _____		**Mission Regional Hospital**

Date	Time	Nurse's Notes

Figure 7.1 Nurse's note.

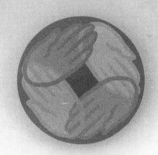

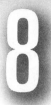

Ethnic, Cultural, and Spiritual Aspects of Care

Name: _____

Date: _____

Course: _____

Instructor: _____

Part 1. Key Terms Review

Match the following Key Term(s) or italicized words from your text with the correct description.

_____ 1. Discrimination

_____ 2. Cultural competence

_____ 3. Prejudice

_____ 4. Culture

_____ 5. Cultural diversity

_____ 6. Stereotyping

_____ 7. Ethnicity

_____ 8. Transcultural nursing

_____ 9. Religion

_____ 10. Spirituality

a. A way of life that distinguishes a particular group of people from other groups

b. Differences between groups of people in a certain geographical area such as a country or medical community

c. Looking at a person or group with preconceived ideas; may lead to mistreatment

d. Formal structured system of beliefs, values, rituals, and practices of a person or group based on teachings of a spiritual leader

e. Care that crosses cultural boundaries or combines elements of more than one culture

f. A determination or judgment about a person or group based on irrational suspicion or hatred of a particular group, race, or religion

g. Type of unfair treatment of one or more persons as a result of misguided beliefs about the person's race, gender, ethnicity, or religious beliefs

h. Choosing to be aware of and familiarize oneself with aspects of cultural differences

i. The categorization of a group of people by a distinctive trait

j. Relationship of the spirit to the body, mind, environment, and other people

Part 2. Connection Questions

Choose the correct answer(s). In some questions, more than one answer is correct. Select all that apply.

11. What item(s) may be worn around the neck of a patient of the Muslim faith?
    a. A replica of the evil eye
    b. A tiny image of Buddha
    c. An amulet containing part of the patient's holy book, the *Koran*
    d. A symbol representing the lion's great spirit
    e. A miniature Brahman

12. Which of the following groups of people always use the right hand to eat?
    a. Amish
    b. Jewish
    c. Asian
    d. Islam
    e. Hindu

13. What of the following is(are) not restricted from the diet by the Jewish culture?
    a. A fish with scales
    b. Pork chops
    c. Beef cooked with milk in a casserole
    d. Eggs and ham
    e. Birds that are predatory in nature

14. Which of the following groups of people may not follow medically restrictive diets because of the belief that it is sinful to refuse what is offered to eat by family or friends?
    a. Native Americans
    b. Asian Americans
    c. African Americans
    d. Hindus
    e. Christian Scientists

15. Which of the following religious groups believe in reincarnation?
    a. Buddhism
    b. Judaism
    c. Amish
    d. Hinduism

16. Because coffee and tea are so commonly served in hospitals, it is important for you to know which cultures forbid or avoid caffeine, coffee, or tea. Which of the following statement(s) is(are) true?
    a. Seventh-day Adventist members are forbidden to consume caffeine.
    b. Some Christian Science members do not believe in consuming coffee or tea.
    c. Latter Day Saints are prohibited from consuming coffee and tea.
    d. Some Asian American groups do not believe in consuming coffee.

17. Which of the following organizations helped establish standards that promote the rights of patients to receive spiritually sensitive care?
    a. The Joint Commission
    b. North American Nursing Diagnosis Association
    c. American Nurses Association
    d. American Association of Nurse Practitioners

18. Which of the following interventions would not be appropriate to assist a patient for whom you have identified spiritual distress?
    a. Use therapeutic communication techniques to encourage expression of feelings.
    b. Allow the patient plenty of opportunities to express his or her feelings.
    c. Teach the patient how your religious beliefs will help the patient to feel better.
    d. Offer presence.
    e. Spend adequate time with the patient, and pay attention to his or her actions, responses, and affects.
    f. Encourage the patient by telling him or her that he or she need not feel abandoned.

Part 3. Review Questions

Indicate whether the following statements are True (T) or False (F).

19. _____ Research studies found that there is no relationship between an individual's religious beliefs or practices and his or her health.

20. _____ If a priest is not available, it is acceptable for you to baptize the dying newborn of Catholic parents if requested by the parents.

21. _____ All cultures have one thing in common: They all believe that they should pray for healing and recovery.

22. _____ The nurse must be aware that coining, a method of treatment for fever, may leave marks on a child that can be mistaken for child abuse.

23. _____ Only when no Muslim community member can be contacted may the health-care providers perform the procedures of preparing the body after death.

24. _____ The nurse must show respect for the patient's beliefs about health care and promote good health practices.

25. _____ A Shaman is utilized for healing by Seventh-day Adventists.

26. _____ Most Buddhists believe that killing of animals for use as a food source is acceptable.

27. _____ Some Native Americans wear amulets to ward off bad spirits or improve health.

Part 4. Application and Critical Thinking Questions

Write a brief answer to the following questions.

28. Mr. Allah is a Hindu and you know Hindus have restrictions of certain foods. What are the traditional dietary restrictions, and what types of food could be offered to him while a patient?

_____

_____

_____

29. What are your own prejudices that you will have to overcome? Include at least one thing you are going to do to overcome one of your prejudices.

_____

_____

_____

30. List three to four barriers related to culture and explain how they can hinder access to health care.

_____

_____

_____

Choose the correct answer(s). In some questions, more than one answer is correct. Select all that apply.

31. When the death of a patient of the Catholic religion appears to be imminent, you will want to consult with the family inquiring if they desire to perform which of the following?
    a. Call a rabbi to administer Communion.
    b. Position the bed toward Mecca.
    c. Call a priest to administer Last Rites.
    d. Notify the Chevra Kadisha so he will be prepared to perform postmortem rituals.
    e. Call a shaman to perform spiritual rituals.

32. Which of the following religious groups forbids blood transfusions?
    a. Jewish
    b. Catholic
    c. Nondenominationalism
    d. Jehovah's Witness
    e. Latter-day Saints (Mormons)

33. Which religious group believes that Allah has all knowledge and control over everything?
    a. Hinduism
    b. Buddhism
    c. Islam
    d. Nondenominationalism
    e. Judaism

Documentation Exercise

▶ *Scenario: Question 34 refers to this scenario.*

The date is March 9, 2017, and you are working 7 p.m. to 7 a.m. on a medical-surgical floor at a rural hospital. It is 2025 (8:25 p.m.) and you have just admitted a 42-year-old male to your floor from the emergency department where he has been since 1655 (4:55 p.m.). He tells you that he has not eaten since lunch and is "starving." Dietary services are closed for the day, but you may have access to some things that he can eat and tell him you will get him something. When you assess his dietary needs, you collect the following nutritional data:

Culture: Asian American
Religion: Buddhist
Allergies: Walnuts and tomatoes
Dietary preference: Vegetarian
Does not eat beef or pork. Coffee and alcohol are forbidden. Eats 5-6 small meals per day. Does drink milk and eat dairy products. Does not eat fish, poultry, or wild game. Likes to have chocolate milk and something sweet at bedtime.
Favorite foods: Vegetarian pizza, egg rolls, baked potatoes, eggs cooked in every way possible, peanut butter, yogurt, dry cereal, peaches, oranges, and bananas.

Checking the physician's orders, you find that he has a regular diet ordered. You proceed to prepare a tray of food for him using the types of foods you might have access to in the unit's nutrition room.

34. Write a narrative nurse's note using Figure 8-1, including the pertinent nutritional data from the data collection. Include an entry documenting what you provided the patient to eat.

Patient _____		
ID# _____ RM _____		
BD _____-_____-_____		**Mission Regional Hospital**
Admit _____-_____-_____		
Physician _____		

Date	Time	Nurse's Notes

Figure 8.1 Nurse's note.

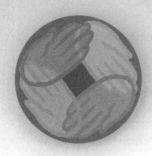

Growth and Development Throughout the Life Span

Name:	
Date:	
Course:	
Instructor:	

Part 1. Key Terms Review

Match the following Key Term(s) or italicized words from your text with the correct description.

_____ 1. Ambivalent

_____ 2. Attachment

_____ 3. Cephalocaudal

_____ 4. Development

_____ 5. Fontanels

_____ 6. Growth

_____ 7. Menarche

_____ 8. Proximodistal

_____ 9. Puberty

_____10. Reflexes

_____11. Regression

a. Spaces between the bones of the skull that have not yet fused

b. Time in which sexual characteristics and function appear

c. Having opposing feelings at the same time

d. Physical changes that occur in the size of the human body

e. Bonding

f. Returning to earlier behaviors, especially in times of stress

g. The increase in complexity of skills performed by a person and/or behavior acquisition that includes walking, talking, and meeting psychological benchmarks

h. Growth that progresses in an orderly fashion from the head downward

i. Onset of menstrual periods

j. Growth that occurs from the center of the body outward

k. Automatic responses by the central nervous system

Human beings grow and develop in different ways over the entire life span. Identify the realms in which people grow and develop by filling in the blanks in the following sentences with the correct Key Term(s) or italicized words from your text.

12. _____ refers to how we learn and was investigated by Jean Piaget.

13. Developing a system that differentiates right from wrong is part of our _____.

14. A person's growing sense of faith is part of their

_____.

15. Genetics, nutrition, the endocrine system, and the nervous system all influence our _____.

16. Eric Erikson defined several stages of our

_____,

which require that we master certain tasks before we can move to the next stage.

Part 2. Connection Questions

Choose the correct answer(s). In some questions, more than one answer is correct. Select all that apply.

17. One of the changes in home health and long-term care is that
    a. Treatment time for older adults is much shorter than it used to be.
    b. Patient populations in home and long-term care have shifted from mostly older adults to patients of all ages.
    c. Hospitals keep patients longer than before so less home care is needed.
    d. Home health and long-term care are carried out primarily by unlicensed aides.

18. A young mother is discussing her twin 2½-year-old toddlers. She says, "It's so cute. They like to run away and play hide and seek when we're in the department store." What does her comment suggest to you, as a nurse, about her needs for education?
    a. This is typical behavior for that age and no particular instruction is needed.
    b. This is typical behavior for that age and the mom should be encouraged to play hide and seek with them.
    c. This is atypical behavior and the mother is probably being inattentive.
    d. The mom needs to be taught about the children's developmental stage and the potential hazards associated with that stage, such as getting lost.

19. Your patient is a 12-year-old girl, admitted for an emergency appendectomy. She is 2 days postop and will be discharged the following day as long as there is no sign of wound infection. You have delegated the responsibility for her care to another nurse, who helps the patient with all aspects of her morning care. You know that yesterday the patient was able to do most of it herself. You ask the nurse about it. Which of the following possible answers represents a developmentally and psychologically appropriate answer for the nurse's actions?
    a. "She didn't seem to want to do it so, of course, I helped her."
    b. "She told me she is afraid of hospitals and was very scared by all the noises last night. She seemed to be regressing a bit, so I determined that she needed extra support today."
    c. "Her mother told me that the little girl needed help with everything."
    d. "She acted like she couldn't do it."

20. You work on a pediatric unit and are caring for a 3-year-old boy who needs to have laboratory work done. What actions should you take if the child starts to panic?
    a. Hold the child firmly and tell him, "Be a big boy. This will hurt a little, but only for a minute."
    b. Show him an instructional storybook about children having procedures done that involve needles.
    c. Speak to the child in a soothing tone of voice. Say, "This may sting a little, but look over here at this book and you won't even feel it."
    d. Speak soothingly to him while distracting him with a toy. Provide comfort immediately after the procedure.

21. You are caring for a 48-year-old woman with ovarian cancer. She has been through surgery and chemotherapy and is now in hospice. She says, "Well, I've had a good life." What stage is she in, according to Erikson, despite her age?
    a. Intimacy versus isolation
    b. Initiative versus guilt
    c. Integrity versus despair
    d. Generativity versus stagnation

Part 3. Review Questions

Choose the correct answer(s). In some questions, more than one answer is correct. Select all that apply.

22. Why is it important for nurses to understand growth and developmental stages?
    a. It is helpful in understanding the patient's actions.
    b. It is important background information.
    c. It helps in planning interventions that will result in the best outcomes.
    d. It is important to teach the patient about what developmental stage he or she is in.

23. You are caring for a 2-year-old child whose mother became a crack addict after the child was born. The child was severely neglected. Which of the following statements represents the best description of this child's psychosocial developmental status?
    a. The child is probably still in the first developmental stage: trust versus mistrust.
    b. The child probably does not feel trusting of people and is in the second developmental stage: autonomy versus shame and doubt.
    c. The child is in the second developmental stage: autonomy versus shame and doubt.
    d. The child has passed the age of the first developmental stage but did not reach the milestone of trust; therefore, he will stay in this stage until he can feel trusting.

24. A baby boy is born into a family of five (three siblings and two parents). The family qualifies for food stamps and medical assistance. He has an atrial-septal defect that will be repaired when he is older. His parents are in their late 30s and are very loving and supportive; they do not speak English very well. What factor will have the most influence on the baby's development?
    a. His heart defect
    b. His loving, supportive environment
    c. His family's lack of extra income
    d. His parents' inability to speak English fluently

Match the stage, according to Erikson, to the appropriate age range.

Stage

_____25. Industry vs. inferiority

_____26. Integrity vs. despair

_____27. Identity vs. role confusion

_____28. Intimacy vs. isolation

_____29. Initiative vs. guilt

_____30. Trust vs. mistrust

Age

a. Birth to 18 months
b. 18 months to 3 years
c. 3 years to 6 years
d. 6 years to 12 years
e. 12 years to 18 years
f. 18 years to 30 years
g. 30 years to 60 years
h. 65+ years

_____31. Generativity vs. stagnation

_____32. Autonomy vs. shame/doubt

Match the task for a stage (presented in order), according to Erikson, to the nursing action that supports the individual in each stage.

Task

_____33. Learn to trust others

_____34. Learn self-control and the ability to express oneself and cooperate

_____35. Initiate activities and influence environment

_____36. Develop sense of social skills and self-esteem

_____37. Seek sense of self and plan according to one's abilities

_____38. Develop intimate relationships and choose career

_____39. Become a productive member of society and establish a family

_____40. Accept worth, uniqueness, and death

Nursing Implication

a. Recognize accomplishments and provide emotional support
b. Keep realistic expectations for behavior and recognize accomplishments
c. Review accomplishments made by the person
d. Increase independence; provide praise and encouragement
e. Avoid criticizing relationships; teach how to establish realistic goals
f. Provide consistent affectionate care
g. Encourage creativity, answer questions; do not threaten or label behavior as "bad"
h. Assist with planning for future and help with decision making

Choose the correct answer(s). In some questions, more than one answer is correct. Select all that apply.

41. Based on Piaget's stages of cognitive development, at which stage would it be best to teach algebra?
a. Formal operational
b. Preoperational
c. Sensorimotor
d. Concrete operational

42. People may not achieve all the stages of moral development and Fowler's stages of spiritual development may be biased to Western cultures. What is important to take away from the information in your textbook about moral and spiritual development?
a. Development along these lines is erratic.
b. Moral and spiritual development may be influenced by many factors.
c. All people have moral and spiritual aspects to their personalities.
d. It is best to assume that people are morally and spiritually developed.

43. Specific newborn reflexes, such as rooting, sucking, startle, and Babinski, all disappear by what age?
a. 2 months
b. 6 months
c. 9 months
d. 12 months

44. Normal growth patterns suggest that the newborn's head circumference will be how much larger at 1 year?
a. Half again as large
b. Twice as large
c. Two and half times as large
d. Three times as large

45. You are giving a class to new parents. One of them asks what the best way to handle temper tantrums is. Which of the following is your best response?
    a. "Take the child to a quiet place and set firm limits on behaviors."
    b. "Ignore the temper tantrum because it is a developmental stage that the child will get over."
    c. "Hold the child firmly and gently tell him or her to stop."
    d. "Reason with the child that temper tantrums will not get the child's desired result."

46. Object permanence refers to the concept that
    a. People can go away and not be seen again.
    b. An object not in the child's sight still exists somewhere else.
    c. Actions have consequences.
    d. Fine motor skills develop after large motor skills.

47. A preschooler who sees his or her parent dressed as Frankenstein will most likely
    a. Think it is funny.
    b. Recognize that it is the parent.
    c. Be frightened.
    d. Not be concerned one way or the other.

48. Question 47 is based on which of the following theories about child development?
    a. Erikson's stage of trust versus mistrust
    b. Kohlberg's stage of individualism and relativism
    c. Piaget's preoperational stage of cognitive development
    d. Fowler's intuitive projective stage

49. Which of the following are characteristics of a 10- to 12-year-old child?
    a. Understands different views about faith
    b. Develops a sense of concern for others
    c. Develops social skills and self-esteem
    d. Understands religion through symbols and stories

50. Puberty is defined as
    a. the stage in which children become interested in the opposite sex.
    b. the stage in which peers become all-important.
    c. the stage in which secondary sexual characteristics develop.
    d. the stage in which dramatic growth spurts occur.

51. You are the school nurse in a large high school. A female student comes to you and asks you about the signs and symptoms of various sexually transmitted diseases (STDs). Which of the following is the best response?
    a. Let the teenager know you are shocked that she needs to ask these questions.
    b. Refer her to different brochures and resources about STDs.
    c. Answer her questions and ask her if she is concerned that she may have an STD.
    d. Ask her what symptoms she is having and reassure that they are probably not signs of an STD. This will gain her trust.

52. One of the most important health-care interventions for toddlers is
    a. Preventing diabetes.
    b. Preventing accidents.
    c. Establishing good bowel habits.
    d. Establishing good hygiene habits.

53. You are counseling new parents and one mother says her 2-year-old will only eat strawberries and chicken fingers. Which of the following is the best response?
    a. "Your child can get all the nutrition she needs from a few foods. Don't worry. She'll eat enough to stay healthy."
    b. "Give her juice and milk to drink to supplement her calories."
    c. "In addition to her favorites, have healthy finger foods available frequently. She'll end up eating enough to stay healthy."
    d. "Have her sit down to a meal. Tell her you will give her strawberries only after she eats her other food. It's important to establish that you are responsible for her nutrition."

Match the following physiological changes that occur in middle age to the clinical manifestation.

_____54. Loss of blood vessel elasticity

_____55. Slower gastric motility

_____56. Loss of subcutaneous tissue

_____57. Decreased production of estrogen

_____58. Decreased production of testosterone

a. Menopause
b. High blood pressure
c. Decreased sperm production
d. Constipation
e. Skin wrinkling

Indicate whether the following statements are True (T) or False (F).

_____59. Young adults generally have few health concerns.

_____60. Lifestyle choices are important for disease prevention.

_____61. Older adults experience a decline in long-term memory as a result of the normal aging process.

_____62. Learning abilities decline in older adults.

_____63. Older adults tend to evaluate their lives more than younger adults.

_____64. Falls are a safety concern for toddlers and older adults.

_____65. Older adults may have bruises and bone fractures as a normal part of aging.

_____66. Young adults should get flu and pneumonia vaccines yearly.

_____67. Unfortunately, confused older adults frequently must be restrained if they are likely to fall and injure themselves. This is because there are no real alternatives.

Match Kohlberg's stages of moral development with their descriptions.

_____68. Punishment and obedience orientation

_____69. Individualism and relativism

_____70. Seeking strong interpersonal relationships

_____71. Law and order orientation

_____72. Social rules and legal orientation

_____73. Universal ethical principles

a. Young adolescent focuses on being good and helping others, not just to follow the rules but to feel good about motives
b. Adult's behavior is motivated by the desire to follow internal values and moral principles
c. Child equates doing right with no punishment and doing wrong with punishment
d. Young adolescent follows laws for the greater good and because of respect for authority
e. Adult has concern for human rights and dignity; desires impartial interpretation of justice
f. Child focuses on what is fair rather than what might be best for the larger group

Fill in the ages and focus for each level of Kohlberg's moral development theory.

Pre-conventional Level

74. Age: _____

75. Focus: _____

_____

Conventional Level

76. Age: _____

77. Focus: _____

_____

Post-conventional Level

78. Age: _____

79. Focus: _____

_____

Part 4. Application and Critical Thinking Questions

Write a brief answer to the following questions.

80. What would be good topics for health seminars for teens, adults, and older adults?

_____

_____

_____

_____

_____

_____

81. Safety is an important consideration for all age groups. Name four specific safety interventions parents can make for their children and apply them to the correct age group. List at least one intervention for preschoolers, school-aged children, and teenagers.

_____

_____

_____

_____

_____

_____

82. Using Erikson's stages of development as a frame of reference, what psychological effect do you think having a serious illness would have on a teenager? How would it be different from the effect a serious illness would have on an adult in his or her mid-30s?

_____

_____

_____

_____

_____

83. Discuss the impact of a serious health crisis for an adult aged 50 years. What physical, psychosocial, and cognitive factors might influence the patient's well-being?

_____

_____

_____

_____

_____

Documentation Exercise

▶ *Scenario: Question 84 refers to this scenario.*

On January 17, 2017, you are caring for a 42-year-old female patient named Juanita Sanchez. Her birth date is 4-19-1974 and her ID # is 364972. She is in Room 302. She was admitted January 13, 2017 for a hypertensive crisis. Her blood pressure was brought under control and she will be discharged on valsartan (Diovan) 160 mg once daily and hydrochlorothiazide 25 mg once daily. While in the hospital, it was discovered that her cholesterol level is mildly elevated at 217 mg/dL. She is 5 feet 3 inches tall and weighs 181 lbs. She works from home doing data entry so she can be home for her three children, ages 3, 6, and 12 years. She is to go home on a healthy heart diet and with orders to walk for 30 minutes a day 5 days per week.

Her mother also lives with the family, but she is on hospice care related to end-stage breast cancer. Mrs. Sanchez is anxious to get home to care for her mother and children. Mr. Sanchez works the night shift. You meet with Mr. and Mrs. Sanchez at 1015 and perform discharge teaching. When you return at 1050, Mrs. Sanchez states that her 12-year-old daughter is having trouble dealing with the impending death of her grandmother. Mrs. Sanchez is also upset knowing that her mother has only a few more months to live. She says she thinks her blood pressure was up as a result of the stress of caring for her mother and from her diet and lack of exercise. She begins to cry, stating that she feels overwhelmed with her mother's care. You discuss the hospice services she is receiving and bring up the possibility of additional help. Mr. Sanchez says that he would be willing to pay for help but does not know how to hire trained, reliable nursing assistants. You offer to arrange a consultation with their current hospice agency regarding more assistance for them. You make the call after leaving the room, at 1115.

84. Document this situation on the nurse's notes (Fig. 9-1).

| Patient _____ |
| ID# _____ RM _____ |
| BD _____-_____-_____ |
| Admit _____-_____-_____ |
| Physician _____ |

Mission Regional Hospital

Date	Time	Nurse's Notes

Figure 9.1 Nurse's note.

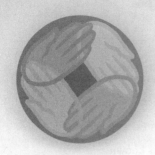

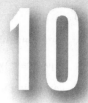
Loss, Grief, and Dying

Name:	_____
Date:	_____
Course:	_____
Instructor:	_____

Part 1. Key Terms Review

Match the following Key Term(s) or italicized words from your text with the correct description.

_____ 1. Apnea

_____ 2. Living will

_____ 3. Postmortem care

_____ 4. Circumoral cyanosis

_____ 5. Advance directive

_____ 6. Role reversal

_____ 7. Comorbidity

_____ 8. Euthanasia

_____ 9. Mottling

_____ 10. Palliative care

a. Cyanosis around the mouth

b. To knowingly administer an unsafe dosage of medication for the purpose of ending the patient's life

c. Pallor of mouth, hands, and feet

d. A specific document indicating what the patient does and does not want medically done should an end-of-life event occur

e. A type of document in which a competent individual can make known any end-of-life wishes regarding medical care (two specific documents fall under this category)

f. A period of no respirations

g. Patches of varying colors of pallor and cyanosis in the feet, legs, hands, and dependent areas of the body

h. Having multiple diseases

i. Comfort care that does not cure the disease

j. Children become the caregivers of their parents

k. The care provided to the body after death

Fill in the blank with the correct Key Term(s) or italicized words from your text.

11. To make arrangements for provision of care so that the family members may have a time to get away, rest, and rejuvenate without the strain and worry of continual caregiving is known as _____.

12. The mental and emotional distress and suffering that one experiences with death and loss are known as _____.

13. An order written by the patient's physician meaning that, should the patient's heart and respirations cease, no cardiopulmonary resuscitation or other efforts to restart the heart and breathing should be performed is called a _____.

14. A legal court document that grants the authority, usually to a relative or trusted friend, to make health-care decisions and act as proxy for the patient should the patient become disabled is known as a

_____.

15. The type of care not intended to cure the patient's disease but is available to assist the patient and family during the last months of life of the patient is known as _____.

Part 2. Connection Questions

Choose the correct answer(s). In some questions, more than one answer is correct. Select all that apply.

16. A female patient in the active phase of dying of lung and bone cancer is dyspneic and her respiratory rate is 10 breaths per minute. She is moaning and cries out when touched or repositioned. Occasionally she cries out without tactile stimulus. Which of the following interventions is most important?
    a. Administer medication to relieve her pain.
    b. Apply oxygen for her dyspnea.
    c. Instruct the staff to avoid repositioning her and leave her supine.
    d. Massage her feet or back to comfort her.

17. A male patient was diagnosed with advanced pancreatic cancer 3 weeks ago and is deteriorating rapidly. Which of the following takes priority?
    a. Make certain the family knows the patient is not doing well.
    b. Talk to the patient about adding chemotherapy treatment to improve prognosis.
    c. Make certain that hospice care has been initiated.
    d. Provide curative care.

18. A living will can establish the individual's wishes regarding which of the following?
    a. Whether a feeding tube may be placed if the individual becomes disabled or an end-of-life condition should occur
    b. Who has the authority to act as proxy for the individual if the individual becomes disabled
    c. Whether the individual may be placed on a ventilator if the individual stops breathing
    d. Which procedures and medications the individual wants if the individual becomes disabled or an end-of-life condition should occur

19. CPR is indicated in which of the following situations?
    a. A patient in the end stages of a terminal disease goes into cardiac arrest.
    b. An individual walking down the street falls to the sidewalk and has no respirations or pulse.
    c. A patient's heart stops when he is in the hospital with severe coronary artery disease.
    d. A patient has been receiving hospice care for 4 weeks.

20. Which of the following cancer survivors may experience a "loss"?
    a. A patient who had a cancerous tumor removed from a kidney
    b. A patient who had a malignant tumor removed from a lung
    c. A patient who had surgical removal of the lower left leg
    d. A patient who had a mastectomy

21. All of the following statements except for one accurately describe changes an individual in the terminal stages of dying may experience with relation to eating. Which one does not?
    a. Food is not needed for the tasks the body now faces.
    b. As death nears, the patient may lose interest in eating.
    c. A patient nearing death may better accept liquids than solid food.
    d. More nutrients are needed to sustain the dying individual.

22. Which of the following should not be taught as a way in which the family can nurture the patient who is getting closer to death?
    a. Encouraging the patient to eat more to keep up strength
    b. Reading a Bible or other religious text to the patient
    c. Sitting close to the patient and reminiscing about memories of fun times they had together
    d. Softly singing one of the patient's favorite songs or hymns
    e. Gently brushing the patient's hair
    f. Gently applying lotion to the patient's feet or hands

23. Your patient has cancer that has metastasized to the bone. You know to monitor the patient for signs of hypercalcemia. Which of the following may be indicative of hypercalcemia?
    a. Confusion, polyuria, lethargy, and vomiting
    b. Increased bone pain, nausea, and fever
    c. Nausea, vomiting, diarrhea, and rash
    d. Dyspnea, bone pain, and restlessness

Indicate whether the following statements are True (T) or False (F).

24. _____ When caring for a dying patient, it is important to ensure that all hands-on nursing care has been completed before taking the time to just sit beside the patient's bed for a few minutes.

25. _____ A patient who is dying and wants to talk about it will always tell you when he or she is ready to discuss the dying process.

Part 3. Review Questions

Choose the correct answer(s). In some questions, more than one answer is correct. Select all that apply.

26. When administering postmortem care, which of the following statements would be true?
    a. There is no need to replace the soiled gown with a clean one because the patient is already deceased.
    b. If an autopsy is to be done, you should remove all tubes and place them in a bag to be sent to the medical examiner for testing.
    c. You should close the eyelids and the mouth, propping the chin with a rolled washcloth if needed.
    d. You should place the body in supine position with the head of the bed flat and the upper extremities positioned next to the sides of the body.
    e. You should make certain that the family is not in the room while administering the postmortem bath.

27. As you are walking down the hall, you pass the door of a room in which there is a woman who is dying of advanced cancer and is nonresponsive. You overhear two women in the room apparently arguing about who should inherit their mother's wedding ring. Based on the fact that hearing is thought to be the last sense to go before an individual dies, you go back and knock on the door of the room where the two women are having the heated discussion. On entering the room, which of the following actions would be the most appropriate?
    a. In a firm voice, tell the two women that hearing is the last sense to go and that they should be ashamed of themselves for discussing this issue in front of their mother.
    b. Ask the women if they need anything.
    c. Assess the patient's comfort and straighten her linens. Then ask the two women if you might speak to them privately.
    d. Enter the room and tell the women that even though visiting hours are not over, that they should leave to allow the patient to rest.

28. When caring for terminal patients and their families, being a good listener involves which of the following?
    a. Taking note of what is—and is not—said
    b. Always listening rather than speaking to the patient and family when you are in the room
    c. Keeping in mind the typical and possible needs, anxieties, and fears that each may experience while conversing with the patient or the patient's family
    d. Being available to listen if the subject matter sounds interesting

Part 4. Application and Critical Thinking Questions

Choose the correct answer(s). In some questions, more than one answer is correct. Select all that apply.

29. Which of the following promises would be appropriate to make to the patient who is dying?
    a. "I promise that you will not be afraid as you get closer to death."
    b. "You will not have any pain or shortness of breath when you die."
    c. "You will die in your sleep and not even know when it is going to happen."
    d. "We will give you medications to control your pain and keep you comfortable."

30. Your patient who is in the end stages of liver failure appears to be speaking to his mother, who you know is deceased. Which of the following describes your best response?
    a. Reorient the patient, reminding him that his mother is deceased.
    b. Allow the patient to talk and do not attempt to correct the patient.
    c. Explain to the patient that there is no one else in the room except you and the patient.
    d. Ask the patient if he believes he is able to communicate with the dead.
    e. Attempt to change the subject to refocus the patient on other things.

31. A patient who is dying is taking very few oral fluids. The patient's son voices concern to you about the lack of fluids and expresses the fear that his father is suffering because he is dehydrated. Which of the following responses would be most important for you to make?
    a. "Let's call the physician and see if he will order some IV fluids for your dad."
    b. "It is believed that dehydration helps to decrease the patient's pain."
    c. "Dehydration decreases production of gastric fluids, which helps decrease nausea."
    d. "Would you like to ask the physician if she would place a feeding tube?"

32. Your patient is a 67-year-old male who is in the advanced stages of cirrhosis of the liver. He has been seriously ill and unable to care for himself for many months. His wife and only daughter refuse to admit him to a long-term care facility and have been caring for him at home 24 hours a day for more than 5 months and are exhausted. He is receiving only palliative care. Which of the following issues is most important to be addressed at this time?
    a. Determine why appropriate treatment is not being administered to cure the cirrhosis.
    b. Ask the physician how long the patient is expected to live.
    c. Help to arrange respite for the patient's wife and daughter.
    d. Evaluate the level of palliative care being provided.

Situation Questions

▶ *Scenario: Question 33 refers to this scenario.*

You are providing care for a 31-year-old female who is in the terminal stages of brain cancer. She is very weak and has periods of confusion. She is mother to three young daughters, ages 2, 5, and 8 years. Her husband has a job that requires him to travel 2 to 3 weeks out of every month. Her parents are deceased. As you finish administering one of her routine medications, she asks you if you have children.

Write a brief answer to the following questions.

33. What should be your next action? Explain your answer.

_____

_____

_____

34. Explain why at the end of a patient's life you should depend less on laboratory values and measurement of vital signs than you do on your skills of observation.

_____

_____

_____

35. Explain what is meant by *giving presence* and why it is so important.

_____

_____

_____

_____

36. How do you personally feel about do-not-resuscitate (DNR) orders?

_____

_____

_____

37. Do you personally believe it is possible to *die well*? Explain your answer.

_____

_____

_____

38. Do you personally believe that each life is significant? Explain your answer.

_____

_____

_____

Documentation Exercise

▶ *Scenario: Question 39 refers to this scenario.*

Date is 7-9-17. Patient is Polie May, an 81-year-old male.

At 0840, Polie May, who is in the hospital receiving chemotherapy for advanced cancer, tells you that he has decided to stop all chemotherapy. He relates that he would rather enjoy a higher quality of life even if it is shorter than to feel constantly sick, weak, and nauseated from the chemotherapy that might buy him only a few extra weeks of time.

He tells you that he discussed it at length with his physician about 2 weeks ago and told the physician that he would let him know when he was ready to discontinue the treatments. After a brief discussion with the patient, you obtain a do-not-resuscitate (DNR) consent form for the patient to sign. You sign the form as a witness of the patient's signature. You tell the patient that if he would like to talk further about anything to please feel free to call you and that you will notify his physician when she arrives this morning for rounds. You then make a copy of the DNR form and provide the patient with a copy, place the original in the patient's chart, and write an entry in the nurse's notes in the patient's chart and on the Kardex and care plan according to facility policy. When his physician arrives at 0930, you inform her of the patient's decision.

39. Document the scenario in the nurse's note form (Fig. 10-1) using the narrative format.

Patient _____		
ID# _____ RM _____		
BD _____ - _____ - _____		**Mission Regional Hospital**
Admit _____ - _____ - _____		
Physician _____		

Date	Time	Nurse's Notes

Figure 10.1 Nurse's note.

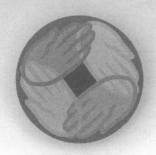

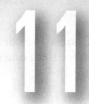

Complementary and Alternative Medicine

Name:
Date:
Course:
Instructor:

Part 1. Key Terms Review

Match the following Key Term(s) or italicized words from your text with the correct description.

_____ 1. Holism

_____ 2. Alternative therapy

_____ 3. Allopathic medicine

_____ 4. Meridians

_____ 5. Complementary therapy

a. Therapy used instead of conventional treatment
b. Energy pathways in the body
c. Therapy used with conventional treatment
d. Relationships among all living things
e. Term used to describe traditional medicine, conventional medicine, or Western medicine

Fill in the blank with the correct Key Term(s) or italicized words from your text.

6. A term used to describe the use of Western medicine and complementary and alternative medicine (CAM) in a coordinated way is _____.

7. The type of CAM named with a combination of two Greek words that mean "done by hand" is _____.

8. _____ is the application of stroking, pressure, friction, and kneading to muscles and other soft tissue to relax muscles and decrease stress.

9. The ancient practice of inserting fine needles into carefully selected points along meridians of the body is called _____.

10. A mind–body intervention used to decrease the negative effects of stress through the use of breathing exercises, physical postures, and mediation is called _____.

11. _____ is a blend of acupuncture and pressure that is a part of traditional Chinese medicine.

Part 2. Connection Questions

Choose the correct answer(s). In some questions, more than one answer is correct. Select all that apply.

12. If you are caring for a patient who uses a type of CAM that is unfamiliar to you, what action will you take?
    a. Ignore the patient's use of CAM.
    b. Change the subject if the patient brings up his or her use of this type of CAM.
    c. Document the patient's CAM use, describing it as an unknown type of CAM.
    d. Ask the patient to tell you more about the CAM that he or she uses.
    e. Avoid showing disapproval of the patient so he or she will feel comfortable sharing information with you.

13. What can be the result of pressure on a spinal nerve by vertebra or other structures?
    a. The patient will experience back pain, numbness, and tingling.
    b. The muscles and organs that the nerve innervates are at risk for dysfunction.
    c. The patient will be paralyzed below the level of the nerve under pressure.
    d. All of these can result from pressure on a spinal nerve.

14. How are the roles of nurses and massage therapists similar?
    a. Both improve the patient's health and well-being.
    b. Both have the opportunity to teach patients about their health.
    c. Both can diagnose medical conditions.
    d. Both focus on relaxing, soothing, and stretching muscles.

15. One of your patients is diagnosed with inoperable lung cancer. He tells you that he had been seeing a massage therapist twice per month. What would you advise him about this use of CAM?
    a. Tell the patient not to have any more massages because it could spread his cancer throughout his body.
    b. Tell the patient to advise his massage therapist about his lung cancer diagnosis because the therapist might need to make changes in what he or she does.
    c. Tell the patient that his doctor will not want him to continue having massages.
    d. Say nothing to the patient about his use of a massage therapist because it is not part of your nursing care.

16. Why is it important to be nonjudgmental when you care for patients who use CAM?
    a. You can learn new things from your patients if you are willing to listen.
    b. You may have the opportunity to teach your patients about potential interactions of CAM use and their medical treatments.
    c. Your patients are more likely to confide in you if they believe that you are not judging them.
    d. All of these are important reasons not to judge patients who use CAM.

Part 3. Review Questions

Choose the correct answer(s). In some questions, more than one answer is correct. Select all that apply.

17. What theory of Descartes affected the way Western medicine and treatments for the mind and the body were developed?
    a. The theory that the mind and body are not connected
    b. The theory that the person's ego controls all aspects of the mind and body
    c. The theory that wellness of the body will bring about wellness of the mind
    d. The theory that all illness, both physical and mental, is controlled by the mind

18. Which of these beliefs is emphasized in holistic health care?
    a. One major factor, such as a bacterium or a virus, is the cause of disease or illness.
    b. Patients should place themselves in the physician's hands to be helped or healed.
    c. Interaction occurs between the mind, body, and spirit.
    d. Each individual is unique.

19. True holistic health care includes
    a. Touching the patient to promote healing.
    b. Reading the aura, or energy, of a person to determine illness.
    c. CAM and Western medicine working together.
    d. Diagnostic and laboratory tests to confirm all diagnoses.

20. Which is true of alternative therapy?
    a. It has not been proved to be effective through scientific testing.
    b. The term is often used interchangeably with complementary therapy.
    c. There is no difference between it and complementary therapies.
    d. It is different from conventional therapies used by the standard medical community.

21. A patient from India is discussing the view of illness and disease in his country. He describes them as
    a. Deviation from normal, healthy body function.
    b. A sign that the person is dwelling on evil thoughts.
    c. The absence of symptoms such as pain or fever.
    d. Caused by an imbalance in bioenergy.

22. What is the focus of a CAM practitioner?
    a. Removing and relieving symptoms
    b. Treating the cause of the illness
    c. Treating diseases diagnosed by laboratory tests
    d. Encouraging prevention of illnesses

23. You and another student are discussing chiropractic. The other student makes all of the following statements about the tenets of chiropractic. Which would you question?
    a. The body is seen as having the potential to correct itself when the nervous system is working at its full potential.
    b. Improving nutrition and lifestyle factors can improve health.
    c. The nervous system is seen as having a major role in health and disease.
    d. It focuses mainly on flexibility of joints, stretching of muscles, and relaxation.

24. A chiropractor would be a good CAM choice to treat
    a. Headaches, joint pain, neck pain, and back pain.
    b. Ulcers, irritable bowel syndrome, and constipation.
    c. Heart disease, diabetes, and hypertension.
    d. Arthritis, tendonitis, sprains, and strains.

25. A patient with which condition(s) might need modification of chiropractic treatment?
    a. Previous back surgery
    b. Scoliosis
    c. Osteoporosis
    d. Arthritis

26. A client comes to a massage therapist with severe osteoporosis. The massage therapist might
    a. Require the client to take a calcium supplement before having a massage.
    b. Massage the client's arms and legs only.
    c. Avoid the use of vigorous or deep massage to prevent injury.
    d. Suggest that the client talk to his or her physician before proceeding with the massage.

27. Which is true of acupuncture?
    a. Its benefits have never been tested or proved.
    b. It is based on classical Chinese medicine.
    c. It involves needles being placed just below the surface of the skin.
    d. It has been endorsed by the National Institutes of Health to treat specific conditions.

28. You are caring for a patient who both practices and teaches yoga. She explains the benefits by citing which of the following?
    a. Yoga realigns the spine and restores function to spinal nerves.
    b. Yoga is believed to balance the mind, body, and spirit.
    c. Yoga practitioners believe it can prevent illness by keeping energy meridians open and flowing.
    d. Yoga is an exercise program designed to build muscle using weights and resistance.

29. A friend is interested in starting a yoga class. She asks you which one would be fast paced and not boring, but where she could easily learn the routine. Based on your knowledge of yoga, which would you recommend?
    a. Power yoga
    b. Iyengar yoga
    c. Hatha yoga
    d. Ashtanga yoga

30. A patient tells you that he sees a massage therapist once a month. He describes his massages as focusing mainly on his feet and says that the therapist often tells him when he has something wrong in his body, even when he has had no symptoms. He is most likely describing which type of massage?
    a. Deep-tissue massage
    b. Swedish relaxation massage
    c. Reflexology
    d. Shiatsu Japanese massage

31. A patient is talking with you about herbal supplements. She shows you a list of all the herbs that she takes regularly and those she takes only occasionally. You look carefully at the list. Which one(s) would you be concerned about her taking?
    a. More than 1 g of ginger
    b. Ephedra
    c. Kava
    d. St. John's wort
    e. Echinacea
    f. Comfrey

32. Which type of CAM involves the use of monitoring devices?
    a. Relaxation and imagery
    b. Meditation
    c. Biofeedback
    d. Therapeutic touch

33. A patient tells you that she manages the stresses resulting from her chronic illness by focusing on a vase of flowers and blocking out all other thoughts to clear her mind. She is describing which type of CAM?
    a. Relaxation therapy and imagery
    b. Meditation
    c. Therapeutic touch
    d. Biofeedback

34. While in the intensive care waiting room with family members, you see a volunteer bring in a large black dog. The dog moves from person to person in the room allowing them to pet him. What are the benefits of this?
    a. Visits from animals can help decrease depression and loneliness.
    b. Petting an animal provides a momentary distraction from anxiety, but it is very brief.
    c. Petting a dog lowers blood pressure.
    d. Animal-assisted therapy may have benefits for a few people, but it is not likely that many people benefit from it.

35. A 4-year-old boy has been traumatized by witnessing the shooting death of his mother by his father. He speaks very little and is unable to verbalize his feelings. Which type of CAM may be helpful for him?
    a. Phytonutrients
    b. Yoga
    c. Biofeedback
    d. Play therapy

Match the following herbs with their uses.

_____36. Gingko

_____37. Saw palmetto

_____38. Echinacea

_____39. Aloe vera

_____40. Garlic

_____41. Valerian

_____42. Soy

_____43. Capsaicin

_____44. Peppermint

_____45. Ginseng

a. A well-known herb that is used alone and in many skin products
b. Used to treat osteoarthritis, fibromyalgia, diabetic neuropathy, and shingles
c. Used as an antiviral agent to prevent or eliminate colds and flu
d. Helps reduce total blood cholesterol and bad cholesterol over 4 to 12 weeks
e. Used for memory enhancement and to treat dementia
f. Used to help lower bad cholesterol and lower blood sugar in type 2 diabetes
g. Used to treat irritable bowel syndrome and decrease intestinal spasms before and after endoscopic procedures
h. Used to treat mild-to-moderate depression
i. Used to treat enlarged prostate in men and to improve symptoms of difficult urination
j. Helps decrease cholesterol and low-density lipoproteins and to treat hot flashes
k. Used to treat insomnia and decrease the amount of time it takes to fall asleep

Part 4. Application and Critical Thinking Questions

Write a brief answer to the following questions.

46. A patient tells you that he uses CAM because he does not like to be a passive partner concerning his health. How would CAM help him accomplish this?

_____

_____

_____

_____

47. Explain what is meant by the statement, "Chiropractors remove interference so that the body can heal itself."

_____

_____

_____

_____

48. A patient tells you that seeing a massage therapist has definitely relieved some of the pain she experiences from rheumatoid arthritis. She asks if that can be true, or if it is all in her mind. How will you respond?

_____

_____

_____

_____

49. Discuss at least two reasons for the popularity of herbal supplements in the United States.

_____

_____

_____

_____

50. Discuss the validity of lifestyle change as a way to heal disease. Is it possible or impossible to sustain?

_____

_____

_____

_____

Situation Questions

▶ *Scenario: Questions 51 and 52 refer to this scenario.*

A friend tells you that he does not understand why you would continue to see a CAM practitioner. He says, "Why do you go to this guy over and over again? I go to the doctor if I have symptoms of something, I get a prescription, and then I get well. That's it!"

51. How will you explain the significance of symptoms in Eastern medicine and CAM?

_____

_____

_____

_____

52. How will you explain the view of preventing illness rather than simply treating illness?

_____

_____

_____

_____

Documentation Exercise

On March 14, 2017, you are caring for a 27-year-old female patient named Kelsea Briggs. She was admitted on March 13, 2017. Her birthdate is 4-19-1989 and her ID # is 664990. She is in Room 1112. She is 28 weeks pregnant with her first child and has been experiencing severe upper abdominal pain, thought to be a gallbladder attack. She has had persistent vomiting, which is now relieved. She is still experiencing nausea, however. The medication for nausea that is prescribed does not seem to be helping her. At 1215, you remove her lunch tray of broth and gelatin. She had not eaten any of it. You ask if you can bring her anything else, but she refuses because of nausea. She refuses any other medications because she is concerned that they "could harm the baby." She then tells you that she has asked her husband to notify her chiropractor, who also does acupuncture. She tells you that early in her pregnancy when she had lots of "morning sickness" that she had acupuncture treatments that helped her. She says her chiropractor is willing to come and do acupuncture treatments for her in the hospital to relieve her nausea. You explain that you will have to get it approved by her attending physician, Dr. Moody, and she asks you to do that.

At 1230, you speak with her physician's assistant (PA) on the telephone and relay the patient's wishes. The PA decides he needs to discuss it with the attending physician first. At 1315, the PA calls and gives you an order for the patient to have acupuncture treatments from her chiropractor.

When you arrive in the patient's room, the chiropractor is already at her bedside. He is pleased to hear that the physician has agreed to the treatment and begins to set up to administer acupuncture. You have never seen acupuncture performed and ask to remain in the room. After a 20-minute treatment with 11 acupuncture needles inserted at different points on her body, the patient tells you that the nausea is much better. At 1420, she asks for some fruit juice and gelatin. You obtain it for her and she consumes all of it.

53. Document this situation on the nurse's notes (Fig. 11-1).

Patient _____		
ID# _____ RM _____		Mission Regional Hospital
BD _____-_____-_____		
Admit _____-_____-_____		
Physician _____		

Date	Time	Nurse's Notes

Figure 11.1 Nurse's note.

Nursing Basics

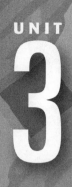

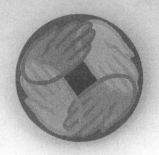

CHAPTER 12

Patient Teaching

Name:	_____
Date:	_____
Course:	_____
Instructor:	_____

Part 1. Key Terms Review

Match the following Key Term(s) or italicized words from your text with the correct description.

_____ 1. Auditory learner

_____ 2. Kinesthetic learner

_____ 3. Visual learner

a. Learning by touching and doing

b. Learning by seeing, reading, and watching

c. Learning by hearing and listening

Fill in the blank with the correct Key Term(s) or italicized words from your text.

4. Teaching patients about getting regular exercise, making healthy food choices, and drinking enough water are examples of _____.

5. Teaching _____ emphasizes changing unhealthy practices.

6. An opportune time to impart information, such as when a patient asks about his or her illness or treatment, is called a _____.

7. When you repeat information several times, you _____ it.

8. When a patient cannot speak English well or at all, it is best to get a(n) _____ when teaching.

9. True _____ occurs when behavior change is the outcome.

Part 2. Connection Questions

Choose the correct answer(s). In some questions, more than one answer is correct. Select all that apply.

10. A 32-year-old male, Mr. Douglas, is admitted for amputation of his left great toe. He will stay overnight in the hospital and be discharged the day after surgery. The toe is very dusky and has a small wound that has not healed in several months. Mr. Douglas developed type 1 diabetes at 19 years of age, and his foot problems are a complication of diabetes. You decide to teach him about his postoperative care before his procedure and then reinforce it later. The preprinted teaching plan gives general information about recovery from anesthesia and provides blank space for individualized teaching points. It is your responsibility to add information about Mr. Douglas's dressing changes and any other specific information you deem important. You think to yourself that Mr. Douglas is fairly young for this complication. Which of the following represents the best nursing judgment about what else should be included in the teaching?
    a. Tell him he needs to take better care of his feet because he will likely end up a double amputee by the time he is 40 if he doesn't.
    b. Tell him to see a certified diabetic educator, and give him some phone numbers to call.
    c. Ask him what he does for foot care and how he manages his diabetes.
    d. Ask him about his family history of diabetes and whether any relatives have had amputations.

11. You work in a pediatrician's office and a 4-year-old girl has several boils that need to be lanced. Which of the following scenarios represents the best teaching plan for the child before the procedure?
    a. Tell her the nurse practitioner is going to fix her boo-boos. Give her some gloves, show her the needle and scalpel, and explain how the nurse will use them. Tell her that she will get the "numbing" needle first and a lollipop afterward.
    b. Tell her the nurse practitioner is going to fix her boo-boos. Take a female doll and draw a few dots on her to represent the boils. Give the little girl gauze, gloves, and a syringe without a needle. Have the little girl don the gloves and clean the area on the doll with an alcohol pad. Tell her to tell the doll that she will feel a little pinch and then have her give the doll the "needle." Let the child use the gauze to clean the dots and then tape a bandage on the doll. Have her give the doll a lollipop.

c. Give the little girl the doll and tell her she can play doctor with it. Let her borrow your stethoscope, give her some tongue blades and other inexpensive supplies, and observe what she does. Note if her play activity involves anything related to the child's health condition.
d. Tell the little girl not to worry, everything will be all right. Explain the procedure but do not show her the needle and scalpel, which will only scare her. Tell her you have to be honest—she will be getting a needle, but the needle will make everything else numb and she will not feel it when the nurse practitioner cleans out her boils. Ask her if she has any questions.

12. You are working on a very busy orthopedic unit. One of your patients, Mr. Godfrey, is being discharged. Much of his teaching has been done; you just have to make sure that he knows how to use his crutches. You are in the room with a new patient who has just arrived from the post-anesthesia care unit when the unlicensed assistive personnel (UAP) tells you Mr. Godfrey is ready to leave. Which of the following represents the best solution for how to handle the demands on your time?
    a. Tell the UAP to check if Mr. Godfrey knows how to use his crutches and that if he does, the aide can escort him to the hospital exit.
    b. Tell the UAP to take over with the postoperative patient while you go and teach Mr. Godfrey to use crutches.
    c. Tell the aide to ask Mr. Godfrey if he would mind waiting for 10 minutes until you can get to see him.
    d. Tell the aide to teach Mr. Godfrey how to use his crutches or to call the physical therapist and ask her to see Mr. Godfrey immediately.

Part 3. Review Questions

Choose the correct answer(s). In some questions, more than one answer is correct. Select all that apply.

13. Which of the following is the best rationale for nurses to perform patient teaching?
    a. Patients are more likely to comply with the treatment plan if they know the purpose and desired effects of the plan.
    b. It saves the doctor time.
    c. None of the other disciplines is responsible for patient teaching.
    d. Patients are less likely to have questions after they are discharged if they are taught everything before leaving the hospital.

14. Which of the following must you assess before making your teaching plan?
    a. The patient's age
    b. The patient's current level of knowledge
    c. The patient's presumed discharge date
    d. The teaching already done by other nurses

15. You have identified a need to teach your patient who has had a skin cancer removed about limiting sun exposure. What is your next step?
    a. Begin telling the patient about the dangers of UV light.
    b. Ask the patient how much time he spends in the sun.
    c. Find resources that discuss his type of cancer and sun exposure.
    d. Tell him to use sunscreen with an SPF of 15.

16. Your nurses' station has handouts about different diseases. What must you determine before giving the handout to a patient?
    a. Is the handout accurate?
    b. Is the handout in the patient's native language?
    c. Is the handout written at about a fifth-grade reading level?
    d. Does the handout have enough illustrations?

Indicate whether the following statements about implementing a teaching plan are True (T) or False (F).

17. _____ Before beginning, establish a comfortable temperature in a room without distractions.

18. _____ Ensure that the patient is in a comfortable position and not experiencing pain or discomfort.

19. _____ Tell the patient to wait until you have finished teaching before asking questions.

20. _____ Adults learn best when they understand the relevance of the information presented.

21. _____ Do not assume an interpreter will be needed. Always ask the patient if he or she wants an interpreter.

22. _____ Speak loudly if the patient wears hearing aids.

23. _____ Present related pieces of information together.

24. _____ Start with the most complicated part of the teaching plan and explain it carefully, gradually reducing it to simple ideas.

25. _____ To help the patient learn a task, ask him or her to try and perform it while you are explaining the correct method.

Choose the correct answer(s). In some questions, more than one answer is correct. Select all that apply.

26. After teaching a patient how to change the dressing on his abdomen, how can you best evaluate his understanding?
    a. Ask the patient to list the first several steps in the procedure.
    b. Ask the patient several questions about the procedure.
    c. Have the patient demonstrate the dressing change for you.
    d. Have the patient explain to his wife how to do the dressing change.

27. A patient is started on a new medication that requires monthly blood tests, and you are teaching her about it. Which response by the patient would indicate the need for more teaching?
    a. "I will have to go to the lab for blood work for as long as I take this medication."
    b. "I can get too much of this medicine in my blood, so I need lab tests to check the levels."
    c. "I may have side effects that I need to tell the doctor about."
    d. "I will go to the lab for a blood test every 6 weeks."

28. After teaching your patient about his diagnosis of congestive heart failure, you ask him questions to be sure he understood the information. This is an example of which of the following?
    a. Assessment
    b. Evaluation
    c. Planning
    d. Implementation

29. Which is an example of appropriate documentation of patient teaching?
    a. "Teaching done on diabetic foot care."
    b. "Instructed on washing and drying feet, inspecting for open or reddened areas, and toenail care by a podiatrist."
    c. "Instructed on washing and drying feet, inspecting for open or reddened areas, and toenail care by a podiatrist. Verbalized understanding and demonstrated correctly."
    d. "Answered questions correctly on appropriate care of feet due to his diabetes. States he will go to a podiatrist to have his toenails clipped."

Part 4. Application and Critical Thinking Questions

Patients will understand a concrete direction more readily than an abstract concept. For example, saying "Sometimes a sodium-restricted diet is ordered for people with hypertension because lowering sodium may lower blood pressure" is more abstract than saying "Do not salt your food at the table. It can cause your blood pressure to go up." Take the following abstract concepts and change them to concrete statements.

30. Safe sex reduces the risk for getting an STD.

    _____

    _____

31. Foods high in saturated fats raise cholesterol.

    _____

    _____

32. Exposure to ultraviolet light increases the risk for getting skin cancer.

    _____

    _____

33. Patient education materials need to be written so that it appeals to the patient. Many different variables, such as the target group's age, can be considered when developing these materials. Taking age into consideration is important because people in the broad age groups (children, young adult, middle aged, and older adult) will recognize themselves in the illustrations and, therefore, be more inclined to believe the information may be of value to them. Think of two other variables to consider and explain why the factor is important to the group.

    _____

    _____

    _____

    _____

    _____

34. Discuss ways in which culture influences health care and patient education.

_____

_____

_____

_____

_____

35. Describe how you would teach a patient who cannot read.

_____

_____

_____

_____

_____

Documentation Exercise

You are caring for Claudia White, a 36-year-old female patient with newly diagnosed diabetes mellitus type 2. She was admitted on April 2, 2017. Her date of birth is 5-14-1980. Her ID # is 2783465 and she is in Room 836. Today is April 4, 2017. You are preparing to teach her how to do finger stick blood sugar testing. At 11:20 a.m., you go to her room to show her how to check her blood sugar before meals. She is anxious and upset, saying that she doesn't like needles and she does not want to "stick" herself. You suggest that she just watch you do the test this time. She relaxes some and pays close attention. You explain each step as you perform it. She tells you that she is surprised that it did not hurt when you used the lancet device to make the puncture on her forearm. You explain that sometimes alternate sites are less painful than using the fingertips. Her blood sugar reading was 145 mg/dL. You explain that normally before a meal, the reading should be between 80 and 120. You also explain that the medication she has been started on will help lower her blood sugar, but that she must also make healthy food choices and avoid concentrated sugars. Ms. White tells you that she knows about diabetic diets because her father had to "watch his sugar" when she was growing up. She said she has some recipes that her mom used to make for her dad.

When you return at 4:30 p.m. to test her blood sugar before the evening meal, you ask if she is ready to try it herself. Although she is nervous and reluctant at first, she is able to "stick" herself on the forearm using the lancet device. She is so surprised that she made the puncture, you have to remind her to insert the strip into the glucometer, then touch it to the drop of blood at the puncture site. She is able to perform the steps, and her blood sugar level is 126. She says she is pleased that it is "closer to what it should be." You tell her what a good job she did and encourage her that she will be able to do this at home. You tell her that, to get even better, she will do her own finger stick blood sugar at bedtime tonight with a different nurse assisting her.

36. Document your patient teaching on the nurse's notes (Fig. 12-1).

Patient		
ID# _____ RM _____		

Mission Regional Hospital

Patient _____
ID# _____ RM _____
BD _____-_____-_____
Admit _____-_____-_____
Physician _____

Date	Time	Nurse's Notes

Figure 12.1 Nurse's note.

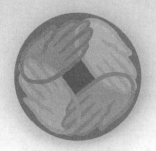

Safety

Name: _____

Date: _____

Course: _____

Instructor: _____

Part 1. Key Terms Review

Match the following Key Term(s) or italicized words from your text with the correct description.

_____ 1. Cardiopulmonary resuscitation (CPR)

_____ 2. Leg monitor

_____ 3. Restraint alternatives

_____ 4. Ambulate

_____ 5. Mass casualty event (MCE)

_____ 6. Rescue breathing

_____ 7. Chair or bed monitor

_____ 8. Heimlich maneuver

a. Walk
b. Pressure-sensitive device that generates an alarm when the patient's weight is no longer sensed
c. Public health or medical emergency that involves thousands of victims
d. Actions to restart the heart or breathing in an unresponsive victim who has no pulse or respirations
e. Breathing for a person in respiratory arrest who still has a pulse
f. A monitor that attaches to the patient and generates an alarm when the leg is in a dependent position
g. Guidelines to help prevent the spread of blood-borne pathogens
h. An action to relieve choking by thrusting just below the xiphoid process
i. Less restrictive ways to help patients remember not to get up or to alert the nursing staff if a patient is attempting to do so

Fill in the blank with the correct Key Term(s) or italicized words from your text.

9. The _____ is the organization responsible for evaluating and accrediting health-care organizations and programs in the United States.

10. A form that gives a numerical rating for each patient's risk for falls is called a _____.

11. _____ are vests, jackets, or bands with connected straps that are tied to the bed, chair, or wheelchair to keep the patient safe.

12. A group of specially trained personnel designated to respond to codes throughout the hospital is the _____.

13. _____ refers to the movement of the muscles of the body for balance and leverage.

14. The middle point of the body, below the umbilicus and above the pubis, around which its mass is distributed is the _____.

15. The _____ refers to the feet and lower legs.

16. A document that contains information about potential harm caused by exposure to a chemical and the directions for what to do if the product gets on your skin or in your eyes or your mouth is called a _____.

Part 2. Connection Questions

Choose the correct answer(s). In some questions, more than one answer is correct. Select all that apply.

17. If you were assigned to care for Mrs. Lloyd, the patient described in the Clinical Connection, which of the following would be your first priority?
    a. Checking the Morse Fall Scale rating for Mrs. Lloyd
    b. Reassuring the family that you will watch her closely so they will not sue the hospital
    c. Assessing risks to her safety and implementing strategies to minimize them
    d. Reading the nurse's notes and care plan to determine how best to transfer her

18. You have delegated the checks and releases of a patient who requires wrist restraints to an unlicensed assistive personnel (UAP). You have been very busy with other patients all morning. The patient's wife finds you and says that her husband is very restless and has not been to the bathroom for 6 hours. What action will you take?
    a. Call the UAP and ask him or her to release the patient and take him to the bathroom.
    b. Go yourself and assess the situation as you release the patient and assist him to the bathroom.
    c. Check the flow sheet, then explain to the wife that the patient has been released every 2 hours and assisted to the bathroom because it is documented.
    d. Call the UAP and question him or her about the checks and releases in front of the patient and his wife.

19. Even if you delegate checks and releases, what are your responsibilities when a patient must be restrained?
    a. Follow up every 2 hours to be sure the patient is released from restraints and has been checked on every 30 minutes.
    b. Remind the UAP every 4 to 6 hours to check on the patient and release him or her.
    c. Avoid delegating any responsibilities related to restraints to avoid legal charges of false imprisonment.
    d. Reassure family members that protocols for restraints are always followed without fail.

20. If you were at a hospital for clinical experience and a mass casualty event (MCE) occurred in your city, how could you and your fellow nursing students be of help?
    a. By leaving the hospital to be out of the way during the disaster response
    b. By taking over all of the staff nurses' responsibilities, leaving them free to respond to the disaster
    c. By participating in the hospital's disaster plan, performing duties as assigned, within your scope as a student
    d. By organizing all of the volunteers who arrive to help during the disaster

21. When injured people come into the hospital after an MCE, if they are unable to provide you with identification, what information can be used to help others identify them?
    a. Hair color
    b. Clothing
    c. Approximate age
    d. Shoe size
    e. Gender

22. When a patient in a home setting uses supplemental oxygen, what teaching should you provide?
    a. No one can smoke in the same room as the oxygen source.
    b. No one can smoke within 50 yards of the house.
    c. No open-flame heaters can be used anywhere in the house.
    d. No candles can be burned in the same room as the oxygen source.
    e. No electrical appliances can be used outside of the kitchen.
    f. Patients using oxygen should not use wool blankets or wear wool sweaters.

23. If a patient who is at risk for falls has a bed or chair alarm in place, you will:
    a. Not need to check on the patient as frequently as you would without the monitor
    b. Instruct the CNA or UAP to turn off the monitor if the patient objects to it
    c. Ask a family member to put on the call light if the patient tries to get up
    d. Check on the patient frequently, ensuring it is in place and turned on

Part 3. Review Questions

Choose the correct answer(s). In some questions, more than one answer is correct. Select all that apply.

24. Before applying restraints to any patient, you must first take which steps?
    a. Try using restraint alternatives without success.
    b. Identify the need for restraints to prevent harm to the patient.
    c. Tell the family that they must watch the patient constantly or else the patient must be tied down.
    d. Ensure that the most restrictive environment is used to prevent harm to the patient.
    e. Obtain a physician's order for the type of restraint and the length of time it is to remain in place.

25. The National Patient Safety Goals are established by what organization?
    a. The Joint Commission
    b. Agency for Health Care Research and Quality (AHRQ)
    c. American Nurses Association (ANA)
    d. Institute for Safe Medicine Practices (ISMP)

26. Hospitalized patients often have impaired mobility causing risk for injury because of what reason(s)?
    a. They are usually old and confused.
    b. They may be weak as a result of surgery or bedrest.
    c. They often have had procedures and tests that cause disorientation.
    d. They all have injuries that cause poor balance.

27. Which of the following factors contribute to an unsafe environment for hospitalized patients?
    a. Age
    b. Impaired mobility
    c. Communication
    d. Pain and discomfort
    e. Prompt assistance
    f. Equipment in the room

28. How are fall assessment scales used?
    a. To predict the number of days a patient will be in the hospital after a fall
    b. To identify patients who have had accidents or injuries during previous hospitalizations
    c. To predict the patient's risk for falls while in the hospital
    d. To serve as reminders to all staff to be aware of safety concerns

Match the restraint alternative to its description. Some answers will be used more than once.

_____29. Pressure-sensitive device generating an alarm when the patient's weight is no longer sensed

_____30. A device that fits across the patient's lap while he or she is sitting in the wheelchair

_____31. Providing backrubs, music, or television as a distraction for a patient who should remain seated or in bed

_____32. Bolsters placed on either side of the patient to prevent entrapment between the side rails

_____33. Keeping the bed at the lowest level at all times except when the staff is at the bedside

_____34. Place an overbed table across the wheelchair like a tray to keep the patient from getting up

_____35. A device that attaches to the patient's upper leg and generates an alarm when the leg is in a dependent position

a. Soft devices
b. Strategies
c. Monitors

Choose the correct answer(s). In some questions, more than one answer is correct. Select all that apply.

36. You walk into a patient's room and discover that he has fallen in the bathroom. What will you do first?
    a. Assist the patient to bed with the help of others, following facility policy.
    b. Notify the physician and explain what happened.
    c. Call for help to get the patient off of the floor.
    d. Check the patient for any obvious injuries, including hip fracture and paralysis.

37. How often must you or an assistant check on a patient who is restrained?
    a. 15 minutes
    b. 30 minutes
    c. 1 hour
    d. 2 hours

38. When a patient is released from wrist restraints, which assessments will you make?
    a. Assess the hands and wrists for edema.
    b. Check capillary refill time in the fingers bilaterally.
    c. Assess the patient's ability to move and feel sensations in the arm and hand.
    d. Assess vital signs.
    e. Assess the skin of the wrists for any open areas.
    f. Assess the patient's orientation to person, place, and time.
    g. Assess the skin under the restraints for redness.

39. What has been a cause of death for patients who were restrained?
    a. The patient tried to get out of the restraint, which caused rapid heart rate and increased blood pressure.
    b. The caregiver physically abused the patient while restrained, which caused blunt trauma.
    c. The restraint was applied incorrectly, which caused choking.
    d. The patient struggled against the restraint, which caused broken skin and overwhelming infection.

40. What must you always do when you apply restraints?
    a. Tie them to the bedrails.
    b. Tie them tightly so the patient cannot struggle.
    c. Administer medications to prevent the patient from being loud or upset.
    d. Tie them in a quick-release knot.

41. If you are in the hospital for clinical experience and you hear "Code Red" called over the intercom followed by a location in another wing of the hospital, what will you do?
    a. Go to the location announced and prepare to help with the emergency.
    b. Close the patient room doors and remain in your area, following facility policy.
    c. Go to the announced location and assist with patient evacuations.
    d. Do nothing because the emergency is not in your area.

42. If you needed to extinguish a fire in the motor of an electric hospital bed, the type of fire extinguisher you obtain would need to be marked with which classification of fire?
    a. Type A
    b. Type B
    c. Type C
    d. Type D
    e. Type K

43. In the event of an MCE, guidelines have been established for shifting standards of care. What do these include?
    a. Treating those most likely to survive first
    b. How to stockpile antibiotics and antivirals
    c. Treating contaminated water to render it safe for drinking
    d. Schedules for calling off-duty staff to work

44. To practice good body mechanics, you would:
    a. Keep the bed in the lowest position while working with patients.
    b. Turn your whole body or pivot on one foot, but avoid twisting.
    c. Bend your knees, not your back, to lift an object from a low shelf.
    d. Carry a heavy object away from your body at waist level.
    e. Avoid pushing or pulling objects; slide or lift them instead.

45. How can nurses avoid being harmed by radiation exposure?
    a. Wear a lead apron during x-ray and fluoroscopy procedures.
    b. Wear a film badge at all times when you work anywhere in a hospital.
    c. If you are pregnant, wear a lead apron at all times during patient care.
    d. Limit the time you spend with patients who have internal or implanted radiation.
    e. Refuse to care for patients who put you at risk for radiation exposure.

Part 4. Application and Critical Thinking Questions

Write a brief answer to the following questions.

46. Why are the elderly more at risk for falls when they are hospitalized?

_____

_____

47. Answering patients' call lights promptly is a safety issue. Defend this statement.

_____

_____

Give the meaning for the following acronyms.

48. What to do if you discover a fire:

    R-_____

    A-_____

    C-_____

    E-_____

49. How to use a fire extinguisher:

P-_____

A-_____

S-_____

S-_____

Situation Questions

▶ *Scenario: Question 50 refers to this scenario.*

You have worked two 16-hour shifts in 4 days and you are very tired. The coworker who was due to relieve you has had a car accident on the way to work. Your supervisor asks you to work another 16-hour shift so he will not have to pull a nurse from another floor who will not be familiar with the patients. You have already worked 8 hours today, for a total of 40 hours this week. You feel that you are too tired to work even another hour, much less 8 more hours.

50. How will you respond?

_____

_____

_____

_____

▶ *Scenario: Question 51 refers to this scenario.*

When you arrive at clinical one morning, you meet a fellow nursing student in the bathroom. She smells of alcohol and is slurring her words. She confides that she was "partying until 4 a.m." and never slept last night. She tells you that she will be fine after a couple of cups of coffee.

51. Do you have any responsibility to share this information? Why or why not? If you do have that responsibility, with whom do you share the information?

_____

_____

_____

_____

52. While assisting with a urology procedure, some Cidex, a strong antiseptic cleanser, splashes into your eye. How will you know the first aid action to take?

_____

_____

_____

_____

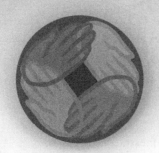

Medical Asepsis and Infection Control

Name: _____	
Date: _____	
Course: _____	
Instructor: _____	

Part 1. Key Terms Review

Match the following Key Term(s) or italicized words from your text with the correct description.

_____ 1. Microorganisms

_____ 2. Pathogens

_____ 3. Health-care–associated infection (HAI)

_____ 4. Primary infection

_____ 5. Localized infection

_____ 6. Septicemia

_____ 7. Medical asepsis

_____ 8. Surgical asepsis

_____ 9. Disinfectant

_____10. Direct contact

a. Infection caused by one pathogen only
b. Microorganisms present and multiplying in the blood
c. Practices performed to prevent the spread of infection; clean technique
d. Cleaning agent that removes most pathogens except some viruses and spore-forming bacteria
e. Minuscule living bodies that cannot be seen without a microscope
f. Method by which microorganisms spread directly from one person to another
g. Free from all microorganisms
h. Microorganisms that cause infection in humans
i. Maintaining a sterile environment, such as that found in the operating room
j. An infection in one area of the body
k. An infection that is acquired while a patient is being cared for in any health-care setting

Fill in the blank with the correct Key Term(s) or italicized words from your text.

11. The tiny plants and animals normally found in the human body are referred to as _____.

12. A _____ is an insect, tick, or mite that spreads infection when it bites humans.

13. The sequence of events that must occur for infection to spread from one person to another is called the _____ of _____.

14. An infection caused by a different pathogen than the primary pathogen is called a _____ infection.

15. A _____ infection is one that spreads through the bloodstream from one site to another.

16. A group of safety measures preformed to prevent the transmission of pathogens found in blood and body fluids is called _____.

17. To prevent the spread of known infection to patients or health-care staff, _____ are used.

18. When you perform procedures in such a way that no pathogens will enter the patient when you insert tubes or give injections, you are using _____.

19. _____ removes all pathogens using steam under pressure, heat, gas, or chemicals.

20. _____ occurs when microorganisms leave one patient and contaminate an object, such as a blood pressure cuff, which is then used on another patient.

Part 2. Connection Questions

Choose the correct answer(s). In some questions, more than one answer is correct. Select all that apply.

21. To protect other patients, yourself, and your family from contagious pathogens such as MRSA, you will:
    a. Wash your hands before and after wearing gloves.
    b. Use standard precautions at all times.
    c. Keep your immune system healthy.
    d. Use transmission-based precautions when indicated.
    e. Use surgical asepsis at all times when caring for patients.
    f. Use hand sanitizer to sterilize your hands after being in a patient's room.

22. When examining a wound drainage specimen under the microscope, you see sphere-shaped microorganisms in chains, appearing similar to a bead necklace. You are looking at:
    a. Staphylococci
    b. Streptococci
    c. Bacilli
    d. Spirilla

23. An antibiotic is described as effective against Gram-positive bacteria. This means that the bacteria:
    a. Appear pink or red after the slide is flooded with Gram stain and rinsed with alcohol
    b. Will not be killed by the antibiotic but will be prevented from multiplying
    c. Appear purple or blue after the slide is flooded with Gram stain and rinsed with alcohol
    d. Are positive for spore-forming characteristics and cannot be killed by any antibiotic

24. Why would emptying the bedside commode be a nursing responsibility rather than a housekeeping responsibility?
    a. Nurses are responsible for doing everything for their patients, including housekeeping tasks.
    b. Nurses are responsible for measuring urine output and creating a pleasant environment for patients.
    c. Nurses can delegate that task to the housekeeping staff, but they must have a doctor's order to do so.
    d. The housekeeping staff should not be expected to perform any task that might put them at risk for contact with blood or body fluids.

25. When teaching a patient how to perform a skill such as administering an insulin injection, be sure to:
    a. Perform the skill repeatedly so the patient will learn how to do it by watching you.
    b. Ask the patient how he or she has seen the injection done by others in the past.
    c. Have the patient try to perform the skill first, then teach the correct way by pointing out his or her errors.
    d. Include instructions on the correct way to perform hand washing in the skill.

26. A patient confides in you that a nurse on a previous shift did not wash her hands before changing the IV bag and tubing. The patient is concerned about this. How will you respond?
    a. "You might want to report her to the head nurse if it happens again."
    b. "It is appropriate for you to ask any health-care worker to perform hand hygiene before touching your tubes."
    c. "I am sure she used hand sanitizer when she came into the room and you just did not see her do it."
    d. "I will talk to her personally and make sure that she knows not to touch you or your tubes without performing hand hygiene."

27. You have delegated the personal care of a patient with *Clostridium difficile (C-diff)* to an unlicensed assistive personnel (UAP). As the supervising nurse, your responsibilities include:
    a. Asking the UAP at the end of the shift if there were any problems caring for the patient
    b. Ensuring that the UAP knows the correct precautions to take to prevent transmission of bacteria
    c. Observing the UAP carefully to ascertain his or her abilities regarding transmission-based precautions
    d. Kindly pointing out any errors in technique to protect the UAP and other patients
    e. Assuming that the UAP will ask if he or she has any questions about transmission-based precautions

Part 3. Review Questions

Choose the correct answer(s). In some questions, more than one answer is correct. Select all that apply.

28. Types of pathogenic organisms include:
    a. Bacteria
    b. Viruses
    c. Vectors
    d. Protozoa
    e. Fungi
    f. Helminths

29. Types of bacteria include:
    a. Helminths and fungi
    b. Cocci, bacilli, and spirilla
    c. Rickettsia and chlamydia
    d. Vectors and protozoa

Match the following pathogens with their descriptions.

_____30. Rickettsia

_____31. Viruses

_____32. Protozoa

_____33. Fungi

_____34. Helminths

_____35. Bacteria

a. One-celled microorganisms classified by their shapes
b. May be made up of one or more cells; enter the human body through cuts or cracks in the skin
c. Rod-shaped bacteria that appear in chains
d. Type of bacteria often spread through vectors
e. Tiny parasites that live within cells of hosts and reproduce there
f. Parasitic worms that can inhabit the digestive tract of humans
g. Single-celled animals that live in water and cause intestinal illnesses when ingested

Choose the correct answer(s). In some questions, more than one answer is correct. Select all that apply.

36. *Streptococcus* type A can cause which of the following illnesses?
    a. Strep throat
    b. Ear infection
    c. Scarlet fever
    d. Gas gangrene
    e. Severe diarrhea
    f. Bloody diarrhea
    g. Heart valve damage

37. Rocky Mountain spotted fever is caused by:
    a. Herpes varicella zoster
    b. *Rickettsia rickettsii*
    c. *Escherichia coli*
    d. *Staphylococcus aureus*

38. Which type of pathogen causes malaria?
    a. Helminths
    b. Herpes simplex
    c. Protozoans
    d. *Candida albicans*

39. A possible cause of a yeast infection resulting from *Candida albicans* is:
    a. Taking antibiotics that kill the normal bacteria in the body, allowing an overgrowth of yeast
    b. That it is a common side effect of taking antifungal medications
    c. The presence of the fungus in food prepared by people with the infection
    d. Consuming undercooked meat that contains the bacteria

40. *Staphylococcus aureus* is the cause of which of the following illnesses?
    a. Toxic shock syndrome
    b. Rheumatic fever
    c. Boils
    d. Necrotizing fasciitis
    e. Osteomyelitis

41. When performing hand hygiene, how much soap do you need?
    a. A pea-sized amount
    b. A dime-sized amount
    c. A quarter-sized amount
    d. Three squirts

42. How can you ensure that you are washing your hands for the correct amount of time?
    a. Count to 20 in your head, saying "one thousand" between each number.
    b. Watch the clock or your watch the entire time you wash your hands.
    c. Tap your foot 20 times while you wash your hands.
    d. Sing "Happy Birthday" twice in your head while you wash your hands.

43. When is it inappropriate to use alcohol gel for hand hygiene?
    a. If you have just come onto the nursing unit to begin your shift
    b. If your hands are visibly soiled
    c. If you have emptied a bedpan or a urinal
    d. If your glove has touched blood or body fluids before you removed it
    e. If it is likely that your hands have been contaminated by spore-forming microbes

Indicate the proper sequence of steps for each procedure.

44. Number in order the steps for donning full personal protective equipment.
    _____ Put on the gown.
    _____ Put on gloves.
    _____ Perform hand hygiene.
    _____ Put on a mask or respirator.
    _____ Put on eye protection.

45. Number in order the steps for removing full personal protective equipment.
    _____ Remove the gown.
    _____ Remove the gloves.
    _____ Remove the mask or respirator.
    _____ Perform hand hygiene.
    _____ Remove eye protection.

Part 4. Application and Critical Thinking Questions

Choose the correct answer(s). In some questions, more than one answer is correct. Select all that apply.

Situation Questions

46. You are removing a feeding pump from the room of a patient who is being discharged. What will you do with the pump?
    a. Put it in the dirty utility room for someone to pick up.
    b. Disinfect it according to facility policy.
    c. Send it home with the patient because he or she has paid for it.
    d. Send it to the Central Supply area of the hospital.
    e. Sterilize it using steam under pressure.

Write a brief answer to the following questions.

47. A patient is diagnosed with "strep throat." Explain how this diagnosis is made, from swabbing the throat to a prescription for antibiotics.

_____

_____

_____

_____

48. Identify all the links in the chain of infection in this situation: A woman becomes ill with pneumonia a few days after sitting next to a man on an airplane for 6 hours. The man was coughing during the entire trip.

_____

_____

_____

_____

49. A fellow student arrives at the hospital for clinical wearing multiple rings with stones on each hand. Why is this a problem for maintaining medical asepsis?

_____

_____

_____

_____

50. You observe a student remove his gloves and leave the patient's room without performing hand hygiene. When you mention it, the student says, "There is no need. I washed my hands and put on gloves. I did not touch anything that was contaminated while in the room. My hands were not dirty." What is your best response?

_____

_____

_____

_____

51. You are planning care for a patient on transmission-based precautions as a result of active tuberculosis. How will you help minimize her feelings of social isolation?

_____

_____

_____

_____

Choose the correct answer(s). In some questions, more than one answer is correct. Select all that apply.

52. A patient has saved her vanilla pudding and milk from her lunch tray. As you assist her with evening care in preparation for bed, the food and drink are still there. When you offer to remove them, the patient says, "No, I might wake up and be a little hungry and eat it tonight." How will you respond?
    a. "That is fine. We can remove it with your breakfast tray in the morning."
    b. "Microorganisms could be growing in it that would make you sick if you eat it."
    c. "If you wake up hungry, push your call light and I will bring you a fresh snack."
    d. "Well, you paid for this food, so you can do whatever you would like with it."

▶ *Scenario: Questions 53 and 54 refer to this scenario.*

A patient is admitted to the hospital after a motorcycle accident. He has many skin abrasions (deep scrapes) and cuts with dirt and gravel embedded in them. This patient also has had diabetes for 10 years. He works two jobs and gets very little sleep. He eats only one meal per day and snacks at night if he has time. After 2 days, he develops reddened, warm areas around the abrasions and cuts. His temperature rises to 102°F (38.9°C), and his white blood count is also elevated.

53. Why is this patient at risk for development of an infection?

_____

_____

_____

_____

54. How is his body attempting to prevent overwhelming infection?

_____

_____

_____

_____

Documentation Exercise

You are caring for a patient with MRSA in a wound who is on contact precautions. At 0730 you provided a bed bath for this patient and assisted her with toileting, oral care, and hair care. You assisted her to the BSC and she voided 650 mL of urine that was clear and yellow. She told you she was lonely and bored. You offered to get her a magazine, and she named one that she wanted. At about 0815 you got the magazine that she requested and brought it to her. You explained to her that the magazine would have to be destroyed when she was no longer on contact precautions, which she said she understood. At 1015, her family came to visit, and you explained to them why she was on contact precautions and how to put on the gown and gloves before entering the room. Then you showed them how to remove the gown and gloves as they left the room at 1130.

55. Document your care and teaching in the nurse's notes (Fig. 14-1).

Patient _____		
ID# _____ RM _____		
BD _____-_____-_____		
Admit _____-_____-_____		
Physician _____		Mission Regional Hospital

Date	Time	Nurse's Notes

Figure 14.1 Nurse's note.

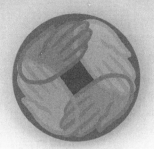

Personal Care

Name:	_____
Date:	_____
Course:	_____
Instructor:	_____

Part 1. Key Terms Review

Match the following Key Term(s) or italicized words from your text with the correct description.

_____ 1. Hygiene

_____ 2. Excoriation

_____ 3. Mottling

_____ 4. Maceration

_____ 5. Vasodilation

_____ 6. Lesions

_____ 7. Lice

_____ 8. Venous return

_____ 9. Leukoplakia

_____10. Seborrhea

a. Softened skin from continuous exposure to moisture

b. Return of blood from the extremities back to the heart

c. Widening of blood vessels

d. White patches on the tongue or oral mucosa that can be precancerous

e. Tiny parasites that live on the scalp

f. Thick, oily scales on the scalp from overproduction of sebum

g. Oil and moisture produced by the sebaceous glands

h. Actions taken to be clean and well groomed

i. Purplish blotching of the skin from greatly slowed circulation

j. Scrapes on the skin

k. Open areas

Fill in the blank with the correct Key Term(s) or italicized words from your text.

11. The preparations for the day, such as bathing, washing and styling hair, brushing and flossing teeth, dressing, and shaving, are referred to as

_____ .

12. Oral care for patients whose conditions result in a need for more frequent care and who need assistance with this care is referred to as

_____ .

13. _____ is a fungal infection that causes a round area of hair loss with a lesion, also called ringworm.

14. _____ are clear bumps affixed tightly to the hair shaft and are the eggs of lice.

15. A custom-made _____ fits the empty eye socket when no implant is in place.

16. A narrow sheet with two narrow hems at each end that is positioned horizontally across the bed, extending from the patient's shoulders to the knees, is called a

_____.

17. A _____ is used to anchor the linens more firmly than if they were only tucked at the foot of the mattress.

18. When a patient needs some assistance with ADLs, the type of care is called _____.

19. When a patient is able to perform ADLs without assistance, the type of care is called _____.

Part 2. Connection Questions

Choose the correct answer(s). In some questions, more than one answer is correct. Select all that apply.

20. If you are assigned to bathe a patient, how should you respond?
    a. Delegate the bath to a UAP or CNA so you can focus on your nursing responsibilities.
    b. Perform the bath as assigned, using it as an opportunity to further assess your patient.
    c. Ask the patient's family if one of them could help the patient bathe because you are very busy.
    d. Wait until nearly the end of your shift before you ask if the patient wants a bath today.

21. What action would you take if you felt that the assignment an instructor has given you is unfair?
    a. Confront the instructor immediately and ask for a clear explanation of why you received such an assignment.
    b. Talk to other students about their assignments and see if anyone else feels the instructor is not fair to them.
    c. Ask to speak to the instructor in private and explain your concerns about the assignment.
    d. Make an appointment to speak with the dean or director of the nursing program to discuss the problem.

22. Which of the following are composed of dead, keratinized cells?
    a. Hair
    b. Sebum
    c. Sweat
    d. Nails

23. The functions of sebum include:
    a. Protecting the skin from cracking and drying
    b. Lubricating the skin
    c. Lowering the body temperature
    d. Evaporating to cool the body
    e. Lubricating hair

24. What causes body odor?
    a. Sebum left on the skin for 24 hours or longer
    b. Bacteria breaking down sweat
    c. The presence of dead, keratinized cells on the body
    d. The presence of sweat in areas that are not open to air, such as armpits

25. How can you ensure privacy for school-age children and adolescents during a bath in the hospital setting?
    a. Stand guard just inside the patient's door to prevent anyone from entering and embarrassing the patient.
    b. Place a "Bath in Progress" sign on the door to prevent interruptions.
    c. Always knock before you enter the patient's room.
    d. Lock the door to the patient's room or bathroom during the bath.

26. Which is true of bathing and caring for the skin of older adults?
    a. Apply lotion frequently to prevent dryness.
    b. Bathe them frequently, 1 to 2 times per day.
    c. Keep the room warm during the bath to prevent chilling.
    d. Sebaceous and sweat glands produce less oil and sweat.

27. If a home health patient is unable to sit down in the bathtub or stand long enough for a shower, what could you do?
    a. Give instructions for the home health aide to perform a bed bath on every visit.
    b. Place a nonrusting lawn chair in the tub or shower and use a sprayer to bathe the patient.
    c. Have the patient sit on a chair near the tub, then use water from the tub to give a partial bath.
    d. Use disinfectant wipes to wash the patient, throwing each one away after using it to cleanse an extremity.

28. If a resident in a long-term care facility has been incontinent but is not scheduled for a bath or shower until tomorrow, what will you do?
    a. Provide perineal care to prevent skin breakdown and odor.
    b. Change incontinent briefs without washing the skin.
    c. Wipe the perineal area with tissue and apply powder to mask any odor.
    d. Change the bathing schedule and give the patient a shower or tub bath now.

29. Under what circumstances would you decide not to delegate a bed bath to a UAP or CNA?
    a. When you need to assess the patient's abilities to participate in personal care
    b. When you need to strengthen the nurse–patient relationship
    c. When you need more information about the patient's skin condition
    d. When the patient's condition is unstable
    e. When the family is present and seems critical of the patient's care

Part 3. Review Questions

Choose the correct answer(s). In some questions, more than one answer is correct. Select all that apply.

30. Which of the following are generally performed as part of morning care (a.m. care)?
    a. Hair care
    b. Bath
    c. Shaving
    d. Oral care
    e. Back massage
    f. Washing hands and face only
    g. Dressing or changing the gown
    h. Straightening or changing linens

31. While you are assisting a patient with a bed bath, you notice a purplish blotching on the skin of the lower legs and feet. This is an indication of:
    a. A reaction to medications
    b. Increased heat in the legs and feet
    c. Infection
    d. Decreased circulation to the legs and feet

32. Your patient is slightly confused. He has activity orders to be up in the chair three times per day. He is unstable on his feet when he walks or stands for more than a few minutes. What type of bath will you plan to give this patient?
    a. Bed bath
    b. Assisted or help bath
    c. Tub bath
    d. Shower

33. It is important to stay with a patient during the first bath or shower after surgery because the patient may:
    a. Be unsteady while standing and sitting
    b. Have an increase in pain when moving about
    c. Cause the incision to open up when getting in the water
    d. Experience vasodilation and become dizzy or faint

34. When you provide oral care to an unconscious patient, you will:
    a. Position the patient on the left or right side with the bed flat
    b. Use lemon glycerin swabs to clean the patient's lips and gums
    c. Assess the mouth for lesions and sores
    d. Use plenty of water to rinse the toothpaste from the teeth and gums
    e. Keep a suction device on and ready for use

35. You are caring for a patient with a nasogastric tube who is unable to take food or fluids by mouth. How often will you perform oral care for this patient?
    a. Oral care is unnecessary because the patient is not eating or drinking anything
    b. Every 2 hours
    c. Every 4 hours
    d. Every 8 hours

36. You are preparing to assist a conscious patient with oral care. The patient has had a stroke, causing partial paralysis of his throat. Once the toothpaste, toothbrush, water, and emesis basin are set up on the overbed table, what will you do?
    a. Instruct the patient to brush her teeth and spit into the emesis basin, then leave the room.
    b. Ask a family member to assist the patient if she needs help while you are out of the room.
    c. Brush the patient's teeth for her, then instruct her to rinse her mouth with water and mouthwash while you prepare for the partial bath.
    d. Stay with the patient in case she chokes while performing oral care, and assist her as needed.

37. When cleaning dentures, you will do which of the following?
    a. Line the sink with a towel or washcloth for a soft surface in case the dentures slip.
    b. Use hot water to rinse the dentures before cleaning them to remove food particles.
    c. Use cool water when washing the dentures to prevent damage to them.
    d. Store them in a denture cup with cool water and a cleaning tablet if the patient wishes.
    e. Clean a partial denture with metal parts by soaking it in water containing a dissolved cleaning tablet.

38. A patient has an IV containing heparin to prevent his blood from clotting. You are assisting him with personal care. Which action will you take?
    a. Shave him with a disposable razor in the direction of hair growth.
    b. Shave him with an electric razor in the direction of hair growth.
    c. Shave him with an electric razor, moving in circular motions over the beard.
    d. Delay shaving this patient until the IV heparin is discontinued.

39. You are providing personal care to a patient with diabetes. Her toenails are a bit long. What will you do?
    a. Do nothing to her toenails because you could cause her to have an infection if you damage her toes.
    b. Clip her toenails carefully straight across but do not file them.
    c. Clip her toenails carefully in a rounded shape to help prevent ingrown toenails.
    d. File her toenails straight across but do not clip them.

40. Your patient has multiple body piercings with jewelry in place. He has been in a motor vehicle accident and is scheduled for an MRI of his left arm and left leg. Which question will you ask this patient?
    a. Do I have your permission to remove the jewelry from your piercings before your MRI?
    b. Are the metals in your jewelry nonmagnetic stainless steel or titanium?
    c. You understand that you will need to remove all of the jewelry from your piercings before you go for an MRI, don't you?
    d. How long has the jewelry in your piercings been in place?

41. Label the following bed positions:
    a.

    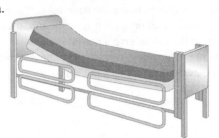

    _____

    b.

    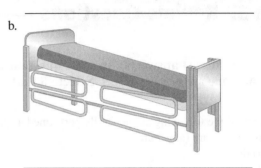

    _____

    c.

    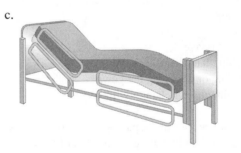

    _____

d.

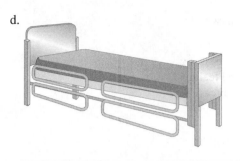

_____

e.

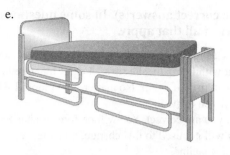

_____

Part 4. Application and Critical Thinking Questions

Write a brief answer to the following questions.

42. What concerns exist about the use of antibacterial soaps?

_____

_____

_____

_____

43. How does giving a bed bath help increase the patient's circulation?

_____

_____

_____

_____

44. Under what circumstances would you omit giving a back massage to a patient?

_____

_____

_____

_____

45. While you are giving mouth care to an unconscious male patient, he keeps biting
down on the sponge stick and toothbrush. What can you do about this problem?

_____

_____

_____

_____

Choose the correct answer(s). In some questions, more than one answer is correct. Select all that apply.

46. You are caring for a patient who has had a left mastectomy. While you are assisting a patient with her bath, she says, "I can't imagine looking in the mirror and feeling good about myself again. No matter how I look, I will still be missing my breast." How will you respond?
    a. "Yes, you are correct. You will be forever changed by this surgery."
    b. "You will get used to this change, and after reconstructive surgery you will be like new again."
    c. "Tell me more about how you feel that your life will be different after this surgery."
    d. "You are worrying more than you need to. No one will know unless you tell them."

Situation Questions

▶ *Scenario: Questions 47 and 48 refer to this scenario.*

You are a male nursing student assigned to care for a female patient from China. She is on bedrest and is experiencing pain and nausea from chemotherapy to treat non-Hodgkin's lymphoma. Communication is difficult and you are not sure if she understands everything that you say. When you ask if she can do her own bed bath, she nods yes. You set up everything for her and leave the room. When you return 45 minutes later, she is asleep and the bathwater looks untouched.

47. What will you do about this situation?

_____

_____

_____

_____

48. Give the rationales for your actions.

_____

_____

_____

_____

Documentation Exercise

You are caring for a 76-year-old male patient with a diagnosis of congestive heart failure and diabetes. His wife tells you that he cannot bathe or shower at home because he gets too short of breath in the shower and cannot get up if he sits down in the bathtub. She tries to help him wash up, but it is difficult for her and him. You teach the patient and his wife ways to conserve his energy during bathing and offer alternatives to standing in the shower or sitting down in the tub.

49. Document your teaching in the nurse's notes (Fig. 15-1). Be sure to include an evaluation of the patient's and his wife's learning.

Patient _____		
ID# _____ RM _____		
BD _____-_____-_____		
Admit _____-_____-_____		
Physician _____		Mission Regional Hospital

Date	Time	Nurse's Notes

Figure 15.1 Nurse's note.

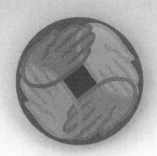

Moving and Positioning Patients

Name:	
Date:	
Course:	
Instructor:	

Part 1. Key Terms Review

Match the following Key Term(s) or italicized words from your text with the correct description.

_____ 1. Plantar flexion

_____ 2. Fowler's position

_____ 3. Dorsiflexion

_____ 4. Semi-Fowler's position

_____ 5. Logroll

_____ 6. Contractures

_____ 7. Lateral position

_____ 8. Transfer

_____ 9. Footdrop

_____ 10. Syncope

a. Permanent plantar flexion of the foot

b. Turn the patient with the body as one unit

c. Move a patient from one place to another

d. Fainting

e. Lying on the right or left side with the back supported, with a pillow between the knees and ankles

f. Sitting position with the head of the bed elevated 30 degrees

g. Ankles flexed at 90 degrees so the toes point to the ceiling when the patient is in a supine position

h. Sitting position with the head of the bed elevated 45 degrees

i. Foot pointing in a downward direction

j. Semi-sitting position with head elevated and knees slightly elevated

k. Shortening or tightening of muscles as a result of disuse

Fill in the blank with the correct Key Term(s) or italicized words from your text.

11. A _____ is placed at the lateral aspect of the patient's thigh to prevent outward rotation of the leg.

12. When a patient's blood pressure decreases with a change in position, it is referred to as _____.

13. _____ occurs when the skin layer is pulled across the muscle and bone in one direction, while the skin slides over the bedsheet in the opposite direction.

14. When you position a patient so that his or her extremities are in alignment to maintain the potential for their use and movement, this is called the _____.

15. The position used to assist patients in severe respiratory distress, allowing maximum expansion of the chest for moving air in and out of the lungs, is called the _____.

16. When you prepare to administer an enema, you will place the patient in the _____ position.

17. The _____ position is described as lying on the stomach with the head turned to the side.

18. The _____ position is described as lying on the back with the arms at the sides.

Part 2. Connection Questions

Choose the correct answer(s). In some questions, more than one answer is correct. Select all that apply.

19. How can you be certain that the wheels of a stretcher are locked before transferring a patient?
    a. Press the foot lock and announce loudly that the wheels are locked.
    b. Physically attempt to move the stretcher, even if you have locked the wheels.
    c. Bend down on one knee to ensure that the red lever is up and the green one is down.
    d. Assign one person to hold the stretcher in place while the patient is transferred.

20. When you care for your assigned patient with paralysis of both legs, you are concerned about skin breakdown. Which nursing interventions would you use?
    a. Reposition him every 4 hours while he is in bed.
    b. Inspect bony prominences for redness every 2 hours. If found, massage around the area but not on it.
    c. Dry skin thoroughly but gently after cleansing it with mild soap.
    d. Pat bony prominences with fluffy towels to relieve pressure points.
    e. Provide adequate nutrition so that the tissue can repair itself.

21. A newly admitted patient with a diagnosis of right-sided weakness resulting from cerebrovascular attack puts on her light and asks for assistance to the bathroom. You have not yet assessed this patient's transfer abilities. What will you do?
    a. Ask the certified nursing assistant (CNA) assigned to the patient to carefully assist her to the bedside commode.
    b. Tell the CNA that the patient has right-sided weakness but can transfer with minimal assistance.
    c. Ask the CNA to accompany you and together transfer the patient to the bedside commode.
    d. Ask the CNA to assist the patient with a bed pan until you have time to get an order for a lift for her.

22. You are concerned about the psychological effects of immobility on the patient you are caring for during your clinical experience. To help prevent psychological complications, you would avoid which of these interventions?
    a. Encourage the patient to stay awake during the day and allow natural light into the room.
    b. Encourage the patient to read, watch TV, solve puzzles, and interact with family and friends.
    c. Encourage the patient to do as much as possible during his personal care.
    d. Encourage the patient to look on the bright side and be glad that he is alive, even though he is paralyzed.

23. Why is it important to explain what you will be doing when you assist a patient with position changes?
    a. The patient may be sedated or have an impaired level of consciousness.
    b. The patient may have a preference about who performs repositioning.
    c. The patient will be more cooperative with the position change.
    d. The patient will be less likely to resist during the position change.
    e. The patient can more easily assist with the position change.

Part 3. Review Questions

Choose the correct answer(s). In some questions, more than one answer is correct. Select all that apply.

24. A patient you are caring for has been on bedrest for 4 days and is having difficulty with gas and constipation. What nursing interventions will you use to help prevent further gastrointestinal complications?
    a. Encourage fluid intake of 6 ounces every 4 hours to prevent further constipation.
    b. Help the patient choose well-balanced meals, keeping in mind the patient's food preferences.
    c. Assess bowel sounds and the frequency of bowel movements, and document.
    d. Serve preferred liquids with a straw to provide continuous access to fluids.
    e. Encourage fresh fruits and vegetable intake, raw if possible, to add fiber.

25. To perform perineal care, you will place the patient in which position?
    a. Dorsal recumbent
    b. Trendelenburg
    c. Reverse Trendelenburg
    d. Sims'

26. Which position will you use for a patient in severe respiratory distress?
    a. Lithotomy
    b. Dorsal recumbent
    c. Orthopneic
    d. Semi-Fowler's

27. When you assist a patient to a left lateral position, where will you place the additional pillows?
    a. Under the knees
    b. Between the knees and ankles and at the back
    c. At the right lateral thigh
    d. At the soles of the feet and at the back

28. You and an unlicensed assistive personnel (UAP) are preparing to turn an immobile patient from her back to her right side. Which of the following actions will you take first?
    a. Place a pillow between her knees and ankles.
    b. Cross the patient's left leg over her right leg.
    c. Move the patient to the left side of the bed.
    d. Externally rotate the patient's right shoulder.

29. When you prepare to turn a patient who has had spinal surgery, you will plan to:
    a. Have a total of three health-care staff assist with the turn.
    b. Have the patient assist by using a trapeze bar.
    c. Have each person turn a section of the patient's body at a separate time.
    d. Logroll the patient.
    e. Have one person at the patient's head to direct the turn.

30. Which assistive device will you use to assist a patient with mild right-sided weakness as he moves from the bed to the wheelchair?
    a. Transfer belt
    b. Slide sheet
    c. Slide board
    d. Transfer board

31. What is the purpose of assisting a patient to dangle?
    a. To increase blood flow to the feet and lower legs
    b. To determine if the patient can tolerate changing positions
    c. To allow time to assist the patient to put on a robe and slippers
    d. To evaluate circulation to all extremities

32. Slide sheets are different from draw sheets because they are:
    a. Placed beneath the patient
    b. Used to move the patient up in the bed
    c. Made of thin webbed nylon
    d. Used to turn the patient from back to side

33. Which assistive device would you use after a patient had fallen to help him or her return to bed?
    a. A slide board
    b. A slide sheet
    c. A transfer belt
    d. A battery-operated lift

34. How will you provide stability as you assist a patient to stand before you begin ambulation?
    a. Place a gait belt around the patient's shoulders.
    b. Place your feet in front of the patient's feet and your knees against the patient's knees.
    c. Have the patient use a walker to stand but not while he or she ambulates.
    d. Place a rolled blanket in front of the patient's feet to prevent slipping.

35. When performing range-of-motion exercises, which action will you take first?
    a. Cover the patient with a bath blanket to preserve dignity and keep the patient warm.
    b. Wash your hands to prevent cross-contamination.
    c. Exercise the patient's neck by moving it from side to side.
    d. Check the patient's chart for any contraindications to full range-of-motion exercises.

Part 4. Application and Critical Thinking Questions

Write a brief answer to the following questions.

36. If a patient is able to bear partial weight but not full weight, which type of assistive device would you select to transfer him from the bed to the wheelchair?

    _____

    _____

    _____

    _____

37. A patient is returning to your unit from surgery. What assistive device would you place in the room prior to the patient's return?

    _____

    _____

    _____

    _____

38. What common linen item might you use to manually transfer a weak patient who is unable to help move herself from a bed to a stretcher, if no assistive devices are available?

_____

_____

_____

_____

Situation Questions

▶ *Scenario: Questions 39 through 41 refer to this scenario.*

You are caring for Mr. Weldon, a patient with a recent cerebrovascular accident (stroke) that has caused right-sided paralysis and affected his speech. He is unable to speak clearly and can only say garbled words. He has orders to be up in the chair bid × 30 minutes. He transfers with the assistance of two staff members. His blood pressure is unstable and sometimes drops more than 30 mm Hg when he stands.

Choose the correct answer(s). In some questions, more than one answer is correct. Select all that apply.

39. Which interventions are appropriate for this patient?
    a. Turn, cough, and deep breathe every 2 hours while in bed.
    b. Perform passive range-of-motion (ROM) exercises to his right side and active ROM exercises to his left side bid.
    c. Avoid positioning him on his right side at any time.
    d. Encourage fluid intake every 1 to 2 hours.
    e. Make decisions for the patient because he is difficult to understand.
    f. Assist him to dangle prior to transferring him to the chair.

Write a brief answer to the following questions.

40. Give the rationale for each intervention that you chose.

_____

_____

_____

_____

41. How will you be able to tell if this patient has pain or discomfort during range-of-motion exercises?

_____

_____

_____

_____

42. Describe a patient who is most at risk for skin breakdown as a result of immobility and being confined to a wheelchair.

_____

_____

_____

_____

_____

_____

_____

43. You are caring for a patient on the first day after surgery. You have orders to get her up in the chair for 30 minutes twice a day. Her BP is 110/64 and P 86 while she is lying down. After you assist her to dangle, her BP is 102/60 and P 102. What will you do?

_____

_____

_____

_____

_____

_____

_____

Documentation Exercise

On January 27, 2017, at 2:45 p.m., as you and a new certified nursing assistant (CNA) attempt to transfer Mr. Weldon from the chair to the bed, his left leg gives way and he begins to fall. You lower him to the floor, but in the process his left arm bumped the chair, causing a 3-inch skin tear. He has no other apparent injuries. His vital signs after the fall are BP 96/60, P 98, and R 22.

44. Describe the actions you will take after you assist Mr. Weldon back to bed.

_____

_____

_____

_____

_____

_____

45. Document what occurred on an incident report (Fig. 16-1) and in the nurse's notes (Fig. 16-2).

Report #_____
Date Received:_____
Initials:_____

Kingfisher Regional Hospital
Unusual Occurrence Report

Date of Event:_____ Time of Event:_____ Department:_____

Patient Last Name:		First Name:		MI
Patient #		Attending Physician:		
Visitor Last Name:		First Name		Phone:
Employee Name:		Dept:		
Physician Name:		Specialty:		

Occurrence Category: (Circle most appropriate)

Fall	Treatment/Procedure	Equipment/Supplies	AMA	Diet Related
HIPAA Compliance	Medication Related	Narcotic Related	Delay in Treatment	Security
Loss of Personal Property	Patient Injury	Order Not Executed	Peer Review Related	Agency Nurse Related
Employee Injury	Visitor Injury	Restraint Related	Other:	

Provide a Brief Description of the Event:

What are the Contributing Factors? (Circle all that apply)

Individual:	System:
Knowledge, Skills, Experience: Unclear or Incomplete	Policies/Procedures Not In Place: Unclear, Outdated
Standard of Care or Practice: Non-Adherence to	Environmental: Staffing, Patient Acuity, Congestion
Documentation: Incomplete or Not Adequate	Communications and Work Flow: Intra & Inter Departmental
	Equipment Failure

Other: (Please Explain)

Submitted by:	Dept.	Date:

Figure 16.1 Incident report form.

Patient _____		
ID# _____ RM _____		
BD _____-_____-_____		
Admit _____-_____-_____		
Physician _____		

Mission Regional Hospital

Date	Time	Nurse's Notes

Figure 16.2 Nurse's note.

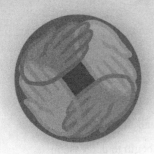

Vital Signs

Name: _____

Date: _____

Course: _____

Instructor: _____

Part 1. Key Terms Review

Match the following Key Term(s) or italicized words from your text with the correct description.

_____ 1. Afebrile

_____ 2. Dyspnea

_____ 3. Orthopnea

_____ 4. Systolic pressure

_____ 5. Bradypnea

_____ 6. Tachycardia

_____ 7. Pulse deficit

_____ 8. Eupnea

_____ 9. Diastolic pressure

_____ 10. Apnea

_____ 11. Bradycardia

_____ 12. Hypoxemia

_____ 13. Stridor

_____ 14. Hypoxia

a. The measurement of the pressure exerted against the walls of the arteries by the blood during relaxation of the heart

b. A high-pitched crowing respiratory sound

c. Respiratory rate greater than 20 per minute

d. Apical heart rate below 60 bpm

e. State of having a fever

f. Apical heart rate is higher than radial pulse rate

g. Having difficulty breathing

h. Inability to breathe without sitting upright

i. Body temperature that is higher than 100°F

j. Decreased level of cellular oxygen

k. The measurement of the pressure exerted against the walls of the arteries by the blood during contraction of the heart

l. When the pulse rate is more than 100 bpm

m. Respirations that are between 12 and 20 per minute, have a regular rhythm, and are of the same depth, neither deep or shallow

n. Without fever

o. A decreased blood level of oxygen

p. A respiratory rate that is less than 12 per minute

q. A period of no respirations

Fill in the blank with the correct Key Term(s) or italicized words from your text.

15. The state of having an elevated body temperature of 102.4°F is known as having a fever. Another term meaning fever is _____.

16. The term used to denote use of a stethoscope to listen to the blood pressure or breath sounds is _____.

17. _____ is the term used to describe a repetitious pattern of respirations that begin shallow, gradually increase in depth and frequency to a peak, then begin to decrease in depth and frequency until slow and shallow, followed by a period of apnea lasting from 10 to 60 seconds.

Part 2. Review Questions

Write a brief answer to the following questions.

18. Describe what is meant by pre-hypertension and include the pressure range to which it refers.

_____

_____

19. List at least eight factors that can affect blood pressure.

_____

_____

_____

20. Describe the difference between cardiac output and stroke volume.

_____

_____

_____

21. Describe the first intervention you should perform when a patient faints because of low blood pressure.

_____

22. To assess the blood pressure on the upper arm, you should place the stethoscope over which artery? _____ Located at which site?

_____

23. What is thermogenesis?

_____

24. What four assessments should you make when assessing respirations?

_____

_____

_____

25. There are a total of six vital signs: five objective and one subjective. Four of the five objective vital signs include the blood pressure, temperature, pulse, and respirations. What is the fifth objective vital sign? _____ The one subjective vital sign is?

_____

Indicate whether the following statements are True (T) or False (F).

26. _____ Based on the circadian rhythm, the body's temperature normally drops 1°F to 2°F in the late afternoon.

27. _____ Antipyretics are medications given for hypertension.

28. _____ When auscultated, the heart sounds should sound muffled and distant.

29. _____ If peripheral pulses can be palpated with each cardiac contraction, the pulses are said to be "perfusing."

30. _____ Hypoxia decreases the pulse rate.

31. _____ If intracranial pressure is increased, the pulse rate will decrease and the BP will increase.

Convert the following temperatures from Fahrenheit to Celsius. Show your work.

32. 100.6°F _____

_____

33. 99.8°F _____

_____

Convert the following temperatures from Celsius to Fahrenheit. Show your work.

34. 37°C _____

_____

35. 40.1°C _____

_____

Choose the correct answer(s). In some questions, more than one answer is correct. Select all that apply.

36. Tidal volume is the measurement of:
   a. The amount of blood contained in a person's vascular system
   b. The volume of blood that is saturated with oxygen
   c. The average amount of air inhaled in one breath
   d. The volume of air exhaled with each breath
   e. The volume of the internal respiration

37. Your patient's BP while sitting was 130/82. Upon standing, the patient became dizzy and her BP dropped to 108/68. This condition is known as which of the following?
   a. Orthostatic hypotension
   b. Secondary hypotension
   c. Pulse pressure hypotension
   d. Postural hypotension
   e. Essential hypotension

38. Which of the following patients have one or more vital signs that are outside normal range?
   a. 28-y/o male with BP 118/76, P 66 regular and strong, R 17, SpO$_2$ 98%, and denies pain or discomfort
   b. 93-y/o female with BP 102/62, P 48 regular and weak, R 22, SpO$_2$ 92%, and denies pain
   c. 15-y/o female with BP 114/68, P 80 regular and strong, R 20, SpO$_2$ 99%, and denies pain or discomfort
   d. Newborn male with AP 174 regular and distinct, R 70, SpO$_2$ 89%

39. The normal range for systolic blood pressure in a healthy 38-y/o adult is:
   a. 100–120 mm Hg
   b. 90–140 mm Hg
   c. 60–90 mm Hg
   d. 100–140 mm Hg
   e. 80–120 mm Hg

Part 3. Connection Questions

Write a brief answer to the following questions.

40. Explain why a person shivers when experiencing hypothermia.

_____

Why does a newborn infant not shiver when the body temperature is below normal?

_____

41. Dehydration decreases the water content of the blood, raising the proportion of red blood cells to plasma, which increases viscosity of the blood. What laboratory test provides the measurement of red blood cell concentration? _____

42. Identify at least two situations in which you should not delegate assessment of vital signs to unlicensed personnel members.

_____

_____

43. Explain why you should not administer aspirin products to children younger than 15 years. _____

_____

44. Mark the eight peripheral pulse sites in correct anatomical locations and identify the pulse site name for each.

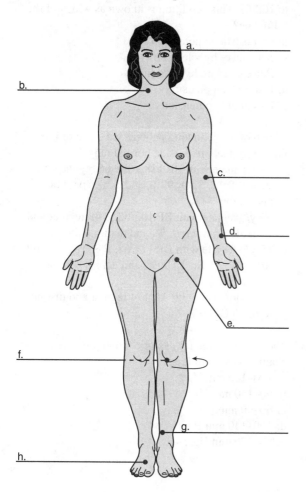

Choose the correct answer(s). In some questions, more than one answer is correct. Select all that apply.

45. Which heart valve(s) close(s) to produce the S_1 sound?
    a. Bicuspid valve
    b. Pulmonary valve
    c. Aortic valve
    d. Tricuspid valve

46. Which part of the central nervous system can affect the rate of heart contractions?
    a. Left temporal lobe
    b. Pons
    c. Hypothalamus
    d. Thalamus
    e. Medulla oblongata
    f. Occiput

47. What characteristic(s) of the pulse should you always assess?
    a. Length of each beat
    b. Strength
    c. Rate
    d. Depth
    e. Rhythm of the beats

48. Which of the following assessments provide data regarding the quality of circulation to a patient's extremities?
    a. Oral temperature
    b. Strength of pedal dorsalis pulse
    c. Skin temperature of hands and feet
    d. Pulse rate
    e. Blood pressure
    f. Color of nailbeds
    g. Capillary refill time

Part 4. Application and Critical Thinking Questions

Write a brief answer to the following questions.

♦ *Scenario: Question 49 refers to this scenario.*

Sheryl Stephens, a 61-y/o female patient who is only a few hours postoperative after having received sedating medication as part of a general anesthesia, presses her call light and requests to get up to the bathroom to urinate. After reviewing the physician's orders to verify that she may get up, you begin to assist her to get out of bed for the first time since surgery. After taking several steps, you notice she is becoming pale as she tells you that she feels like she is going to faint. You assist her immediately back to the bed where you help her to lie down.

49. What do you expect to find on assessing her vital signs? What has she most likely experienced, and what should you do to handle the situation? What might you have done in an attempt to prevent this episode from occurring?

_____

_____

_____

_____

_____

▶ *Scenario: Question 50 refers to this scenario.*

You are caring for Brent Hammond, a 71-y/o male with congestive heart failure. As a result of this disease, his heart's ability to pump blood is markedly decreased, resulting in less cardiac output than normal.

50. When you assess Mr. Hammond's apical pulse, two radial pulses, and two dorsalis pedis pulses, what characteristics of these various pulses might you expect to obtain in your findings?

_____

_____

_____

_____

Documentation Exercise

Document the following data as you would in the nurse's note form using Figure 17-1.

51. On November 7, 2017, at 0700 you assessed your patient's vital signs and found the systolic blood pressure to be 148 and her diastolic pressure to be 94, oral temperature to be 99.8°F, pulse rate to be an irregular but strong 95 beats per minute, and respirations to be 27 breaths per minute. Her oxygen saturation on room air was 98 percent. She complained of pain (6) in her right flank area. You used a pain rating scale of 0 to 10.

| Patient _____ |
| ID# _____ RM _____ |
| BD _____-_____-_____ |
| Admit _____-_____-_____ |
| Physician _____ |

Mission Regional Hospital

Date	Time	Nurse's Notes

Figure 17.1 Nurse's note.

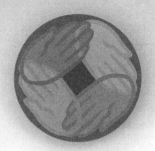

Applying Heat and Cold

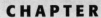
Name: _____	
Date: _____	
Course: _____	
Instructor: _____	

Part 1. Key Terms Review

Match the following Key Term(s) or italicized words from your text with the correct description.

_____ 1. Vasodilation

_____ 2. Phagocytosis

_____ 3. Metabolism

_____ 4. Vasoconstriction

_____ 5. Edema

_____ 6. Hypothermia

_____ 7. Contraindication

a. Chemical and physical processes required to build and maintain body tissues

b. The inner lumen of blood vessel becomes smaller

c. Swelling caused by excessive fluid shifting to the interstitial space

d. A condition in which it is not safe to perform a specific treatment

e. Having excessive intracellular and intravascular fluid

f. White blood cells surround, engulf, and digest microorganisms

g. A body core temperature below 95°F

h. A condition for which a treatment is useful

i. Increase in size of the vessel lumen

Fill in the blank with the correct Key Term(s) or italicized words from your text.

8. When heat packs are left in place longer than 45 minutes, the vessels may constrict rather than dilate. This is known as _____.

9. A device with a small, electrically heated water-storage tank and two tubes connected to a network of tubing within a disposable pad, used for application of heat, is known as a(n) _____.

10. _____ is the term used to describe irregular blotches of pallor and bluish purple discoloration of the skin, a sign indicating that a cold application is too cold.

Part 2. Connection Questions

Choose the correct answer(s). In some questions, more than one answer is correct. Select all that apply.

11. The physiological effects of local heat application include:
    a. Dilation of veins
    b. Constriction of veins
    c. Relaxation of muscle spasms
    d. Decreased blood flow to the area
    e. Increased delivery of oxygen to the area
    f. Increased delivery of nutrients to the area

12. Which of the following physiological changes make the elderly more susceptible to burns from heat applications?
    a. Thinner skin
    b. More porous bones
    c. Reduced tactile sensation
    d. Cognitive changes

13. Patient teaching regarding home use of heating pads should include which of the following?
    a. Use the highest temperature setting for maximum heat penetration.
    b. Set a timer for no longer than 20 to 30 minutes.
    c. Use a thin layer of petroleum jelly on skin to prevent burns.
    d. Use heat on areas that continue to swell.
    e. Never lie on top of a heating pad.
    f. Check the skin under the heating pad every 10 minutes for excessive redness.

14. When using a tepid bath for fever reduction, the longest a child should be left in the tepid water is _____.
    a. 60 minutes
    b. 45 minutes
    c. 30 minutes
    d. 15 minutes

15. When systemic cooling of the body is used in cardio-vascular surgery, what are the effects of the therapy?
    a. Slowed metabolism
    b. Ischemia of cells
    c. Reduction of body's oxygen requirements
    d. Phagocytosis

Write a brief answer to the following question.

16. Which type of heat penetrates the deepest—dry or moist? Explain your answer.

_____

_____

_____

_____

Part 3. Review Questions

Choose the correct answer(s). In some questions, more than one answer is correct. Select all that apply.

17. All of the following, except one, are indications for heat application. Which condition would not be a suitable indication?
    a. Sore muscles after working in the garden for several hours
    b. An infected cut on the plantar surface of the foot
    c. A newly jammed thumb joint
    d. A postoperative patient with a body temperature of 95°F

18. Which of the following physiological changes will help an infected wound to heal?
    a. Phagocytosis
    b. Increased blood flow to tissue
    c. Vasoconstriction
    d. Decreased delivery of oxygen to tissue
    e. Delivery of increased level of nutrients to site
    f. Increase in cellular metabolism

19. Common uses for cold applications include:
   a. Hypothermia
   b. Fever reduction
   c. Pain relief
   d. Hemostasis
   e. Prevention of swelling
   f. Reduction of edema

Write a brief answer to the following questions.

20. Explain the risk associated with administration of a sitz bath.

_____

_____

_____

_____

21. What assessments should you make during local applications of cold therapy?

_____

_____

_____

_____

22. Why must you always place a thin cloth barrier between an ice pack and the patient's skin?

_____

_____

_____

_____

23. How long does it take a local heat application to achieve maximum vessel dilation?

_____

_____

_____

_____

Part 4. Application and Critical Thinking Questions

▶ *Scenario: Questions 24 through 28 pertain to the following scenario.*

Marla, a 51-year-old female, sprained her right ankle approximately 2 hours ago. The ankle exhibits 3+ pitting edema and extensive reddish blue ecchymosis. Marla complains of an aching, burning pain at a 6 on a scale of 0 to 10, with 0 being no pain and 10 being the worst pain she can imagine. She asks if she can put a hot pack on the ankle for comfort.

24. What answer should you provide Marla? Support your answer with details.

_____

_____

_____

25. Should you apply heat or cold at this very early stage of recovery? Which method of application might work best in this situation?

_____

_____

_____

26. What assessments should you make prior to the application?

_____

_____

_____

27. What is the maximum length of time this type of therapy is left in place?

_____

_____

_____

28. What physiological effect will it have on Marla's ankle?

_____

_____

_____

▶ *Scenario: Questions 29 and 30 pertain to the following scenario.*

William May, an 85-year-old male with a chronic musculoskeletal condition, is a resident of a long-term care facility. He suffers severe muscle spasms as a result of the musculoskeletal condition. After lying in bed all night, it is difficult for him to regain flexibility for daytime activities. In an effort to relax his tight muscles, the physician has ordered that Mr. May be given a whirlpool bath, rather than a bed bath, each morning before beginning his daily activities.

29. What risks or concerns should you be aware of prior to assisting Mr. May into a whirlpool bath?

_____

_____

30. What interventions should you perform to prevent these possible problems from occurring?

_____

_____

Documentation Exercise

▶ *Scenario: Question 31 refers to this scenario.*

Marla, a 51-year-old female, sprained her right ankle approximately 2 hours ago. The ankle exhibits 3+ pitting edema and extensive reddish blue ecchymosis. Marla complains of an aching, burning pain at a 6 on a scale of 0 to 10, with 0 being no pain and 10 being the worst pain she can imagine. You apply an ice-filled pack to her ankle. You elevate the ankle on two pillows and make certain to place a towel between the ice pack and her skin. While the cold pack is in place, you assess it every 15 minutes and find the skin cool and pink. She tells you that the pain is somewhat better, down to a 4, after leaving the ice pack on for 30 minutes. After you take off the pack, the skin assessment findings are the same as during treatment.

31. Document the situation and assessment findings prior to treatment, during treatment, and immediately after treatment in the nurse's note form (Fig. 18-1). Include the effectiveness of the cold pack, which is known as the evaluation phase of the nursing process.

Patient _____		
ID# _____ RM _____		Mission Regional Hospital
BD ____-____-____		
Admit ____-____-____		
Physician _____		

Date	Time	Nurse's Notes

Figure 18.1 Nurse's note.

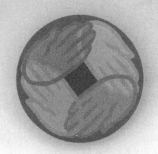

Pain Management, Rest, and Restorative Sleep

Name: _____

Date: _____

Course: _____

Instructor: _____

Part 1. Key Terms Review

Match the following Key Term(s) or italicized words from your text with the correct description.

_____ 1. Acute pain

_____ 2. Cutaneous pain

_____ 3. Chronic pain

_____ 4. Referred pain

_____ 5. Neuropathic pain

_____ 6. Radiating pain

_____ 7. Phantom limb pain

_____ 8. Visceral pain

_____ 9. Intractable pain

_____ 10. Nociceptive pain

a. Stimulation of deep internal pain receptors

b. Pain lasting longer than 6 months

c. More superficial pain of skin and underlying subcutaneous tissue

d. Type of neuropathic pain that feels as though it is coming from an amputated (missing) extremity

e. Pain that cannot be relieved, is incurable, or is resistant to treatment

f. Pain of a duration less than 6 months

g. Pain felt in an area other than where it was produced

h. Pain that originates in the mind

i. Pain caused by stimulation of pain receptors

j. Burning, stabbing, or deep ache caused by nerve compression/damage as a result of pressure from tumors, edema, or compression fractures

k. Pain that begins at a specific site and shoots out from or extends to a larger area beyond the origin site

Fill in the blank with the correct Key Term(s) or italicized words from your text.

11. The view of a patient's pain that includes mental, social, physical, and spiritual aspects as parts of the integrated whole being is known as _____.

12. The process by which drugs may be administered, within preset boundaries, by the patient, who controls the frequency and administration of his or her pain medication, is called _____.

13. Certain pain receptors are randomly dispersed throughout the skin, subcutaneous tissue, and muscular tissue. These nerve pain receptors can be stimulated by temperature changes, tissue damage, and certain chemicals. These receptors are known as _____.

14. The pain receptors referred to in question 13 can be stimulated by two chemicals that are released during injury and damage to tissue. One of those chemicals is

_____.

15. The second chemical that stimulates the pain receptors in question 13 is _____.

16. Classes of medication that either produce pain relief from a mechanism different from traditional analgesics or by potentiating or increasing the effects of opiates, opioids, and nonopioid drugs are known as

_____ drugs.

17. The medical term for pain medications is

_____.

18. Repetitive gentle, gliding stroking of your fingertips over the surface of the skin for the purpose of pain relief is called _____.

19. The natural body chemicals produced by the brain in response to pleasant thoughts or feelings, exercise, laughter, sex, and massage, and that act similarly to morphine and produce feelings of euphoria, well-being, and pleasure are known as _____.

20. That rest that allows an individual to awaken feeling rested, refreshed, rejuvenated, energized, and ready to meet new challenges is _____.

Part 2. Connection Questions

Choose the correct answer(s). In some questions, more than one answer is correct. Select all that apply.

21. Your 98-year-old patient has severe diabetes and, as a result of complications, had his left leg amputated above the knee several months ago. He is confused and combative. When he reports to you that his left foot hurts, you know that this is known as:
    a. Radiating pain
    b. Nonexistent pain
    c. Phantom limb pain
    d. Intractable pain
    e. Chronic pain

22. Which of the following statements is (are) thought to accurately describe the gate control theory?
    a. Transmission of pain impulses to the central nervous system is controlled by a gate that is opened and closed by sensory stimulus.
    b. Stimulation of the broad nerve fibers by heat, cold, massage, and exercise is thought to open the gate, allowing pain impulses to be transmitted.
    c. Stimulation of the smaller, narrow nerve fibers by injury and damage to the tissues is thought to open the gate, allowing pain impulses to be transmitted.
    d. It is thought that the thalamus can open the gate when stress and anxiety increase, and close the gate when stress and anxiety decrease.

23. An individual's thoughts and emotions are also believed to affect the opening and closing of the gate by stimulating production of:
    a. Prostaglandins
    b. Endorphins
    c. Substance P
    d. Opioids

24. Your patient seems to be having a lot more postoperative pain today than he did yesterday, which surprises you because he has been progressing so well since his surgery 4 days ago. As you are critically thinking about factors that can increase pain, you identify data that could explain why he is having an increase in pain today. Which of the following pieces of data might provide you with this understanding?
    a. His wife, who is a strong part of his support system, was here to visit this morning for several hours.
    b. In the report, the night nurse noted that he slept only a couple of hours last night.
    c. His medical chart indicates that he is Native American, a culture in which some feel that pain should be suffered in silence.
    d. Earlier this morning, the patient's wife mentioned that the patient is really missing their oldest daughter, who was unable to come for the surgery because she lives in Europe.

25. Which of the following are types of nociceptive pain?
    a. Cutaneous pain from a paper cut
    b. Soft tissue pain caused by injury to the thigh muscle and subcutaneous tissue
    c. Deep somatic pain from arthritis or a bone fracture
    d. Deep visceral pain from hysterectomy postoperative pain

26. Who is the best judge of the severity of a patient's pain?
    a. The patient who is experiencing the pain
    b. The surgeon who performed the surgery
    c. The nurse who is monitoring the patient
    d. The spouse of the patient who is staying with the patient

27. Which of the following information would be included in a pain assessment?
    a. Characteristics of the pain
    b. Level of the pain
    c. Whether the patient has a low pain tolerance
    d. What the patient wants done for the pain

Write a brief answer to the following questions.

28. You have medicated a female patient for severe pain and are waiting for the medication to take effect. In an effort to relieve her discomfort, you decide to try an additional nonpharmacological intervention. After explaining what you are about to do, you begin to verbally direct the patient to focus her conscious mind on the sequential tightening and relaxing of her muscles, beginning at her head and working toward her feet. What is the medical term for this intervention? How does it work?

_____

_____

_____

29. Briefly describe how various aspects of lifestyle, environmental factors, and stress can affect sleep and rest.

_____

_____

_____

Part 3. Review Questions

Choose the correct answer(s). In some questions, more than one answer is correct. Select all that apply.

30. Because pain slows healing and recovery, relief of pain has become a higher priority while caring for patients. As a result:
    a. Pain has been classified as a vital sign.
    b. Pain should never be allowed to become more painful than a 1 on a scale of 0 to 10.
    c. Pain should be assessed once per shift.
    d. Pain should be assessed every time you assess the vital signs.

31. Your patient reports having severe pain at an 8 on a scale of 0 to 10. You notice that her vital signs are all within normal range. Which of the following statements accurately explains the normal vital signs?
    a. The patient is not really hurting if the blood pressure and pulse are not elevated.
    b. Acute pain does not generally elevate the vital signs.
    c. The body learns to adapt to chronic pain and, therefore, does not elevate the vital signs.
    d. The patient is having nociceptor pain, which does not affect the vital signs.

Fill in the blank with the correct term(s) from the text.

32. The patient usually snores, accompanied by periods of apnea lasting from 10 seconds to 2 minutes; this can be life-threatening. This inability to maintain breathing while sleeping is known as _____.

33. The intolerable crawling sensation in the legs that results in an irresistible urge to move legs is known as _____.

34. Grinding of teeth during sleep is termed _____.

35. A condition that causes uncontrollable, recurrent daytime episodes of sleepiness that can hinder driving and operating dangerous equipment is called _____.

36. The term for chronic inability to fall asleep or stay asleep is _____.

37. Confusion and disorientation in elderly patients that occur in the evening hours is commonly known as _____.

Part 4. Application and Critical Thinking Questions

Choose the correct answer(s). In some questions, more than one answer is correct. Select all that apply.

38. Acetaminophen is a common over-the-counter medication used by most individuals. What is the maximum dose limit for an adult?
    a. Four 250-milligram tablets per 24 hours
    b. Two 500-milligram tablets every 4 hours
    c. 1000 milligrams every 3 to 4 hours, for a maximum of 8000 milligrams per 24 hours
    d. 4000 milligrams per 24 hours

39. The category of drugs that have greater capacity for addiction and abuse is regulated by law. The correct terminology for these drugs is which of the following?
    a. Controlled substances
    b. Prescription drugs
    c. Injectable drugs
    d. Analgesic drugs

40. Common aspirin has more than one classification and is used for different problems. Which of the following is (are) not a classification of aspirin?
    a. Antipyretic
    b. Analgesic
    c. Antihistamine
    d. Antiplatelet
    e. Anti-inflammatory

41. Which of the following drugs are not classified as over the counter?
    a. Ibuprofen
    b. Aspirin
    c. Acetaminophen
    d. Codeinex

42. Which of the following are not classified as controlled substance drugs?
    a. Naproxen
    b. Meperidine
    c. Dilaudid
    d. Morphine
    e. Fentanyl

Write a brief answer to the following questions.

43. Briefly describe two categories of adjuvant drugs and how they work to relieve pain.

_____

_____

_____

_____

_____

_____

44. Describe how the following nonpharmacological methods work to reduce mild pain or to use as an adjuvant (along with pain medication) for more severe pain: guided imagery, effleurage, and a TENS.

_____

_____

_____

_____

_____

_____

45. What are the benefits of using a PCA?

_____

_____

_____

_____

_____

_____

_____

Documentation Exercise

▸ *Scenario:*

Winona Smith is a 73-year-old female with severe fibromyalgia, arthritis, and lupus. She has been admitted for chest pain to rule out angina (cardiac pain that may precede a heart attack). She rings her call light, and when you answer the light, she complains of severe pain.

46. Create a faux pain assessment that contains all of the components you should include. Document the assessment on Figure 19-1, a nurse's note form. Be accurate, thorough, and succinct.

		Mission Regional Hospital
Patient _____ ID# _____ RM _____ BD ____-____-____ Admit ____-____-____ Physician _____		

Date	Time	Nurse's Notes

Figure 19.1 Nurse's note.

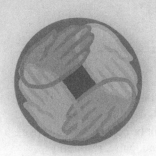

Admission, Transfer, and Discharge

Name:	_____
Date:	_____
Course:	_____
Instructor:	_____

Part 1. Key Terms Review

Match the following Key Term(s) or italicized words from your text with the correct description.

1. Working together with the patient and family to systematically plan how to best meet the patient's needs after hospitalization is the process known as

   _____.

2. When a child or an older adult who is dependent on a caregiver is separated from the caregiver, such as when hospitalized, it can cause severe anxiety and loneliness, which is known as _____.

3. The chart form that is used to list the patient's medications and how to take them, required modifications or restrictions of diet or activity, situations and signs and symptoms that warrant physician notification, and care or treatment that the patient is to continue at home is known as the _____.

4. The form used to document the patient's condition and reason for transfer, and that includes a comprehensive list of the patient's medications is the

   _____.

5. If a patient becomes unhappy with his or her care, decides against treatment, or for any other reason simply decides to leave the hospital before the physician authorizes a discharge, this is known as

   _____.

6. One of the most important things you will do for your patient at discharge is to compare the current list of medications your patient is taking at discharge with the list of medications the patient was taking at home to ensure there are no omissions, duplications, or potential drug-drug interactions. This process is known as

   _____.

Part 2. Connection Questions

Choose the correct answer(s). In some questions, more than one answer is correct. Select all that apply.

7. Simple things that you may do to reduce separation anxiety in a child include:
   a. Encouraging a parent or guardian to stay with the child as much as possible
   b. Asking the parent or guardian to bring a familiar blanket, pillow, or stuffed animal that the child sleeps with at home
   c. Asking the parent or guardian to stay until the child goes to sleep before leaving
   d. Asking the parent or guardian to bring a favorite toy and book from home
   e. Offering to arrange for meals to be sent for the parent at each mealtime

8. Ways to reduce separation anxiety in an older adult might include which of the following?
   a. Providing the patient with a brief but factual explanation of his or her diagnosis and why he or she must be in the hospital
   b. Explaining that visiting hours do not allow someone to stay with an adult
   c. Reassuring the patient whenever possible without giving false reassurance
   d. Allowing a spouse or family member to stay with the patient

9. An RN must assess each patient upon admission to health-care facilities. The source of this requirement is:
   a. The Nurse Practice Act
   b. The facility's policy
   c. The Joint Commission
   d. The admission committee

10. Which of the following statements is (are) accurate regarding the delegation of admission assessment duties?
   a. All of the assessment must be performed by the RN.
   b. Portions of the assessment can be assigned to the LPN/LVN.
   c. The entire assessment can be performed by the LPN/LVN and then signed by the RN.
   d. Some things such as assessment of vital signs, weight, and height may be delegated to unlicensed personnel.

11. Objective components of an initial assessment database would include some, but not all, of the following. Which components would not be considered objective?
   a. Blood pressure, temperature, pulse, respirations, oxygen saturation level
   b. Pain level, location, and characteristics
   c. Level of consciousness
   d. Auscultation of heart, breath, and bowel sounds
   e. Peripheral pulses and capillary refill
   f. Range of motion and strength of all extremities
   g. Weight and height

12. Subjective components of an initial assessment database would include which of the following?
   a. Level of consciousness
   b. Pupillary reaction to light
   c. Whether or not the patient uses illicit drugs
   d. The patient's use of sleep aids, cigarettes, alcohol, and laxatives
   e. The patient's complaints of fatigue, dizziness, and insomnia

13. Discharge planning should begin:
   a. Early morning on the day of discharge
   b. The day before the physician plans to discharge the patient
   c. On admission to the facility
   d. Once the patient begins to improve

14. The patient must be taught about new medications that are to be taken on discharge from the facility. Which of the following statements is (are) accurate about this patient teaching?
   a. Teaching should include as few details as possible to make it easier to remember.
   b. It is not necessary to write down the medication instructions as long as the patient understands what you have told him or her.
   c. The best time to teach the patient about new medications is just before he or she leaves the facility so that the information will still be fresh in his or her mind on arrival at home.
   d. You should ask for clarification that the patient understands the instructions.

15. What subjects should be included in discharge teaching?
    a. When to return to the physician's office for follow-up
    b. List of medications, how to take them, and what side effects to watch for
    c. Required modifications or restrictions of diet or activity level
    d. Signs and symptoms of worsening condition that warrant physician notification
    e. Care or treatment that the patient is to continue at home

16. Which of the following should be included in your last nurse's notes entry at discharge?
    a. The patient's condition
    b. Vitals signs
    c. The time the patient actually leaves
    d. The method of transportation
    e. Notification of housekeeping

17. Some of the following individuals contribute to the discharge plan. Which one(s) would not contribute?
    a. Unlicensed assistant
    b. Occupational therapist
    c. Dietician
    d. Social worker
    e. Nurse

18. Which of the following data would not be appropriate to include on a transfer summary form?
    a. A list of patient's discharge medications
    b. A note describing how difficult it is to get the patient to take medications
    c. Current diet order and activity restrictions
    d. Patient teaching that has been done and the patient's response
    e. Follow-up appointments

Part 3.   Review Questions

Choose the correct answer(s). In some questions, more than one answer is correct. Select all that apply.

19. The time to begin establishing rapport with your patient is:
    a. As soon as you completed the patient admission and carried out admission orders, such as starting an IV
    b. As soon as the patient begins to ask questions about his or her medical problems
    c. The first time you meet the patient during admission
    d. When you go in the room to perform an unpleasant task for the patient

20. Common fears a patient may experience and ask about include:
    a. What is wrong with me?
    b. What tests, procedures, treatments, or surgeries will I undergo?
    c. Under which level of Maslow's hierarchy does this fear fall?
    d. How long will I have to be here?
    e. How much will this cost?
    f. Will I make a good impression on the admission's office staff?

21. Which of the following is (are) not included as part of the admission process?
    a. Eating the diet tray ordered by the physician
    b. Obtaining consent to treat
    c. Application of identification bands
    d. Orienting patient and family to the environment
    e. Transporting the patient to physical therapy

22. You are discharging a patient and have a list of duties to perform to complete this discharge. Which of the following responsibilities is most important?
    a. Notifying the laboratory personnel that the test scheduled for today has been canceled
    b. Assisting the patient to dress in his or her own clothes
    c. Redistributing the patient workload for the staff now that a patient is to be discharged
    d. Reconciling the patient's medications
    e. Noting the physician's order to discharge the patient

23. Which of the following would NOT be a therapeutic nursing intervention that demonstrates respect and compassion for patients' common reactions to admission?
    a. Smiling when meeting a new patient
    b. Explaining what you are doing to do prior to doing it
    c. Encouraging the patient to ask questions
    d. Explaining to the patient that there is no need to be embarrassed when you expose his or her body

Fill in the blank with the correct answer.

24. The discharge process includes notifying the

    _____

    department(s).

25. The loss of control that patients often experience when hospitalized comes under which level of Maslow's hierarchy of patient needs? _____

26. When should you check the patient's ID band?

   _____

27. What is the one intervention you can perform before each nursing task that will increase patient compliance?

   _____

Part 4. Application and Critical Thinking Questions

Choose the correct answer(s). In some questions, more than one answer is correct. Select all that apply.

28. In an effort to decrease the patient's feelings of loss of control, which of the following would be appropriate without compromising provision of appropriate care?
   a. Ask if the patient would prefer to wear a hospital gown or personal sleepwear.
   b. Provide a menu, allowing the patient to select food choices from those available on the prescribed diet.
   c. Ask the patient if he or she prefers to have the IV started in the right or left hand.
   d. Ask the patient if he or she prefers to be NPO or to be on a special diet.
   e. Allow the patient to decide if he or she prefers vital signs to be assessed just once daily or every 4 hours.
   f. Give the patient the choice of taking a shower in the morning or at bedtime.
   g. Allow the nonsurgical female patient to determine whether or not you leave her underwear in place.

29. Which of the following may contribute to a patient's loss of identity?
   a. The patient may feel that he or she is just another patient out of many patients.
   b. The patient does not have identification bands on.
   c. The patient may feel like he or she is just another patient number.
   d. The patient is separated from familiar family members.
   e. The patient may feel that he or she is just another diagnosis.
   f. The patient is of a different culture than the general population of his or her health-care providers.

Write a brief answer to the following questions.

33. You are caring for Sam Wilbanks, a 37-year-old father of four children, who has been hospitalized for a myocardial infarction (heart attack). He tells you that he has no health insurance and cannot miss any further work. To whom should you refer Mr. Wilbanks?

   _____

   _____

   _____

30. Which of the following interventions would help to prevent loss of identity?
   a. Address the patient by his or her surname.
   b. Put the patient's name on all of his or her valuables.
   c. Avoid referring to the patient by his or her room number.
   d. Do not call your patient endearing names such as sweetie pie, dear, or honey.

31. After explaining a test or procedure to the patient, you would observe for both objective and subjective signs of understanding or confusion, which will indicate whether or not your patient teaching was effective. This is known as which phase of the nursing process?
   a. Planning
   b. Diagnosis
   c. Implementation
   d. Evaluation

32. Discharge planning may cover many subjects. Which of the following subjects might be included as part of discharge planning?
   a. Teaching how to perform colostomy irrigation
   b. Providing the patient with a list of available community resources, such as Meals on Wheels or Women, Infant, and Children Services
   c. Providing the family with a list of long-term care facilities that would meet their needs
   d. Making a referral to a home health agency

34. You are caring for a patient who is still quite ill and is not ready for discharge. The patient states, "I have had enough of this place and I'm leaving." Briefly describe your responsibilities in this situation.

_____

_____

_____

_____

_____

_____

35. Discuss at least three reasons a patient may feel "loss of control" when hospitalized, and identify interventions that would be helpful.

_____

_____

_____

_____

_____

_____

_____

_____

_____

_____

_____

_____

_____

_____

36. Lakshanyai Arora is a 35-year-old male patient assigned to you, a female nurse. He is Hindu and relates that his faith requires that his health-care provider be a male, but there are no male nurses working the current 12-hour shift. What types of interventions might you incorporate in an effort to make the best of this situation?

_____

_____

_____

_____

_____

_____

_____

37. Describe the five safety issues you ensure when medication reconciliation is performed.

_____

_____

_____

_____

_____

_____

_____

_____

38. List four reasons for completing an admission orientation checklist.

_____

_____

_____

39. Identify at least four types of data you are responsible for collecting at admission (other than physical assessment).

_____

_____

_____

_____

_____

40. Besides physical assessment of all body systems, what additional physical assessments should you make on admission?

_____

_____

_____

_____

41. Which of the following should be trusted to determine a patient's weight on admission: the patient, your estimation, or the scales?

_____

Why would you think that accuracy would be important?

_____

Documentation Exercises

▶ *Scenario: Questions 42 and 43 refer to this scenario.*

You are admitting a new patient to your floor from the emergency department who is scheduled to go to surgery in approximately 1 hour. He has various valuables with him and there is no family member in attendance who can take the valuables home. The patient tells you that he has the following items that will need to be locked up: an expensive leather wallet made of shark penis skin worth $960 and containing $1300 in $100 bills; a platinum Rolex watch; a 24-karat white-gold wedding band with a 1-karat diamond; a 4G iPhone by Apple that is red; and a black Louis Vuitton iPhone case worth $1100.

42. In the following space, objectively document the items the patient has given to you to secure until his wife arrives late tomorrow night from visiting her family in Zurich.

_____

_____

_____

_____

43. On a nurse's note form (Fig. 20-1), document a faux pain assessment performed during an admission assessment. Include all the necessary components and be accurate, thorough, and succinct.

Patient _____		Mission Regional Hospital
ID# _____ RM _____		
BD _____-_____-_____		
Admit _____-_____-_____		
Physician _____		

Date	Time	Nurse's Notes

Figure 20.1 Nurse's note.

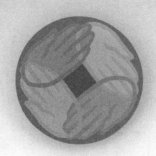

Physical Assessment

Name:	_____
Date:	_____
Course:	_____
Instructor:	_____

Part 1. Key Terms Review

Match the following Key Term(s) or italicized words from your text with the correct description.

_____ 1. Aphasia

_____ 2. Auscultation

_____ 3. Accommodation response

_____ 4. Orthopnea

_____ 5. Excursion

_____ 6. Dysphasia

_____ 7. Jaundice

_____ 8. Ptosis

_____ 9. Retractions

_____10. Sordes

a. Numbness or a decreased sensation

b. Chest wall appears sunken in between the ribs or under the xiphoid process as the patient inhales

c. Patient knows what he wants to say but cannot say the words

d. Yellow or orange coloring of the skin and mucous membranes

e. Listening to the sounds produced by the body

f. Drooping of the eyelid

g. Difficulty coordinating and organizing the words correctly

h. Dried mucus or food caked on the lips and teeth

i. Pupils constrict when focusing on a close object and dilate when focusing on a far object

j. Equal chest expansion during inspiration

k. Difficulty breathing while lying flat

l. Both pupils constrict to the same size and at the same rate when stimulated by light

Fill in the blank with the correct Key Term(s) or italicized words from your text.

11. Use of your four senses allows you to detect evidences of illness or injury. These evidences that you collect, with the exception of something the patient may tell you, provide you with objective data. What are these pieces of objective data called? _____

12. The information that the patient tells you provides you with subjective data that require validation. What are these pieces of subjective data called? _____

13. Application of your hands to the external surfaces of the body to detect abnormalities of the skin or tissues just below the skin is termed _____.

14. The assessment technique of using your middle finger to tap against your other middle finger placed against the patient's body surface is known as _____.

15. Abnormal sounds that can be auscultated over the lung fields are called _____.

16. You have assessed the patient's pupils by shining a light into both pupils as you learned to assess both pupil reflexes and accommodation response. What acronym would you document that would indicate that all findings were within normal parameters? _____

17. During assessment of your patient, you notice that the patient has numbness of the left side of her face. You would use the medical term _____ to document this finding.

18. While assessing the patient's oral mucosa, you detect severely unpleasant sour breath. What is the correct medical terminology for this finding? _____

19. During palpation of the patient's abdomen, he flinches and tightens the abdominal muscles where you are palpating. This tightening of abdominal muscles is known as _____.

20. What medical term would be appropriate to use when reporting that your patient is drowsy or mentally sluggish? _____

Part 2. Connection Questions

Choose the correct answer(s). In some questions, more than one answer is correct. Select all that apply.

21. What type of assessment is performed on admission?
    a. A focused assessment
    b. An initial head-to-toe shift assessment
    c. A comprehensive health assessment
    d. A brief admission systems assessment
    e. Disease and injury assessment

22. A patient was admitted yesterday with pneumonia. When auscultating his breath sounds you detect rales in the right lower lobe. How quickly should you reassess this abnormal finding?
    a. Within 15 minutes
    b. Within 60 minutes
    c. In less than 2 hours
    d. In 4 hours or less
    e. When the patient complains of dyspnea

23. A 5-year-old child has a fever of 104.4°F axillary. When should you reassess the child's temperature?
    a. Within 60 minutes
    b. Within 90 minutes
    c. Within 2 hours
    d. Within 4 hours

24. Which of the following statements applies to the Muslim religious group?
    a. They believe that underwear cannot be removed except in emergency situations.
    b. They tend to be mistrustful of and cautious with nurses and physicians until they know them better.
    c. They are extremely immodest.
    d. They prefer health-care providers of the same gender as the patient.

25. Select the symptom(s) from this list of assessment findings.
    a. Flushing
    b. Fever of 102.8°F
    c. Nausea
    d. Vomiting
    e. Light-headedness
    f. Cramping
    g. Guarding
    h. Hypoactive bowel sounds

26. Blood pressure can provide you with information regarding which of the following?
    a. Central nervous system
    b. Cardiovascular system
    c. Integumentary system
    d. Renal system
    e. Fluid status
    f. Infection

27. Body temperature can provide you with information regarding which of the following?
    a. Central nervous system
    b. Immune system
    c. Hydration level
    d. Infection
    e. Respiratory system
    f. Cardiovascular system

28. Which of the following assessment findings may provide you with neurological status data?
    a. Thick, dirty hair
    b. Lethargy
    c. Color of the lower extremities
    d. Edema of the left hand and arm
    e. Pulse rate of 44 bpm

29. Which of the following can be indicators of a person's hydration level?
    a. Color of nailbeds
    b. Temperature of skin on lower extremities
    c. Sluggish capillary refill
    d. Positive consensual reflex
    e. Weight
    f. Thirst

30. The cone portion of each lung extends approximately 1 inch above the medial aspect of the clavicle and is called what?
    a. Lower lobe
    b. PMI
    c. Bronchus
    d. Apex
    e. Base

31. Which lobe(s) of the lungs is(are) not accessible for auscultation posteriorly?
    a. The left upper lobe
    b. The left lower lobe
    c. The right upper lobe
    d. The right middle lobe
    e. The right lower lobe

32. Which lobe(s) of the lungs is(are) accessible for auscultation only posteriorly and laterally?
    a. The left upper lobe
    b. The left lower lobe
    c. The right upper lobe
    d. The right middle lobe
    e. The right lower lobe

33. Which lobe(s) of the lungs is(are) accessible for auscultation both anteriorly and posteriorly?
    a. The left upper lobe
    b. The left lower lobe
    c. The right upper lobe
    d. The right middle lobe
    e. The right lower lobe

34. The bottom of the lower lobes of the lungs extends down to which of the following?
    a. 8th intercostal space midclavicular line anteriorly
    b. 6th intercostal space laterally
    c. 10th intercostal space anteriorly
    d. 6th intercostal space midclavicular line anteriorly
    e. 8th intercostal space posteriorly
    f. 10th intercostal space laterally

35. You have just completed auscultation of the patient's lungs. The sounds that you heard were sort of rattling; however, they cleared when the patient coughed. What term accurately describes what you heard?
    a. Rales
    b. Rhonchi
    c. Wheezes
    d. Pleural friction rub
    e. Stridor

36. If you hear a shrill, high-pitched, crowing sound coming from the room of a 3-year-old child who has croup, you recognize the ominous sign known as:
    a. Rales
    b. Rhonchi
    c. Wheezes
    d. Pleural friction rub
    e. Stridor

37. At which of the following locations can you best hear the sound of the aortic valve?
    a. Just to the left of the sternum in the 3rd intercostal space
    b. To the left of the sternum in the 5th intercostal space in the midclavicular line
    c. Just to the right of the sternum in the 2nd intercostal space
    d. Just to the right of the sternum in the 4th intercostal space

38. The off-going nurse reported to you that one of your patients had been having an irregular pulse for several hours. You plan to assess this patient's heart rate carefully during your initial patient rounds at the beginning of your shift. Which of the following would be the most accurate way to do this?
    a. Palpate a radial pulse in both wrists for 30 seconds.
    b. Auscultate the apical pulse for 60 seconds.
    c. Take a second nurse with you to palpate the radial pulse at the same time that you auscultate the apical pulse for 60 seconds.
    d. Palpate the PMI for a full minute.

39. You know that when assessing the pulse there is more than one characteristic you should assess. Which of the following best identifies the characteristics you must assess?
    a. Rate, rhythm, and strength
    b. Rate, volume, and strength
    c. Regularity and number of beats per minute
    d. Site of PMI, rate, and strength

40. You are caring for a patient with mitral valve stenosis. You plan to assess the mitral valve during your initial assessment. Where will you be best able to auscultate the mitral valve?
    a. The right base of the heart
    b. The left base of the heart
    c. The apex of the left ventricle
    d. The left lateral sternal border

41. When you assessed the radial pulse and the apical pulse of one of your patients, you noted that one of the pulses was slower than the other one. Which one of the following describes the assessment finding that you obtained?
    a. The radial pulse was faster than the apical pulse.
    b. The apical pulse was faster than the radial pulse.
    c. The radial pulse was slower than the apical pulse.
    d. The apical pulse was slower than the radial pulse.

42. Another nurse working on your floor reports that one of the patients has an apical pulse of 87 bpm and a pulse deficit of 9. You know that means the patient's radial pulse was:
    a. 96 bpm
    b. 87 bpm with 9 skips
    c. 78 bpm
    d. 9 bpm

43. You are preparing to perform an initial shift assessment. You know that the correct order in which you should perform the five techniques for objective assessment (except for the abdomen) is:
    a. Auscultation, olfaction, observation, palpation, and percussion
    b. Observation, auscultation, palpation, percussion, and olfaction
    c. Observation, palpation, percussion, auscultation, and olfaction
    d. Olfaction, auscultation, observation, palpation, and percussion
    e. Olfaction, observation, auscultation, percussion, and palpation

44. The correct sequence to assess the abdomen is:
    a. Auscultation, olfaction, observation, palpation, and percussion
    b. Observation, auscultation, palpation, percussion, and olfaction
    c. Observation, palpation, percussion, auscultation, and olfaction
    d. Olfaction, auscultation, observation, palpation, and percussion
    e. Olfaction, observation, auscultation, percussion, and palpation

45. What are the acronyms used to indicate the quadrants of the abdomen?
    a. RLQ
    b. LMQ
    c. LUQ
    d. RMQ
    e. RUQ
    f. LLQ

46. You have just completed an initial shift assessment of your 72-year-old female patient who has congestive heart failure. Which of the following assessment findings causes you the most concern?
    a. Fine papular rash under both breasts
    b. Reports her last BM was 2 days ago
    c. AP 78 regular and distant
    d. Has not voided in 12 hours
    e. Complaints of fatigue

47. You have just completed an initial shift assessment of a male in his 30s with a history of elevated hypertension and elevated cholesterol. Which of the following assessment findings provides information about his circulatory system?
    a. Skin is pale, warm, and dry.
    b. BP is 164/98.
    c. R is 27 regular and even.
    d. AP is 94 regular and 2+, RP is 90 irregular and 2+, and pulse deficit is 4.
    e. Pedal pulses are weak and equal bilaterally.
    f. He has 2+ edema of both ankles.
    g. He is awake, alert, and oriented to four spheres.

48. During a focused assessment of a patient's circulatory system, you were unable to palpate the left pedal pulse although the right pedal pulse was strong. What should be your first action?
    a. Notify the physician.
    b. Check the blood pressure in the left leg.
    c. Palpate for the left posterior tibialis pulse.
    d. Obtain a Doppler.

49. Which of the following would be the most accurate description of dorsal flexion assessment?
    a. Ask the patient to press his or her toes toward the foot of the bed, applying pressure against the palms of your hands so you can assess the strength and equality of the flexion between the two sides.
    b. Ask the patient to pull his or her toes toward the head, pulling against the palms of your hands so you can assess the strength and equality of the flexion between the two sides.
    c. Ask the patient to gently point his or her toes toward the foot of the bed so you can assess agility and coordination of the lower extremities.
    d. Ask the patient to gently point his or her toes toward the head so you can assess the neuromuscular activity of his lower extremities.

Part 3. Review Questions

Write a brief answer to the following questions.

50. What is the medical terminology for each of the "lubb dupp" heart sounds?

_____

51. Which of the two heart sounds is the loudest? _____

52. List all the assessments that are part of a neurological examination.

_____

_____

_____

_____

Choose the correct answer(s). In some questions, more than one answer is correct. Select all that apply.

53. Which of the following assessment findings is not within the textbook normal range?
    a. 23 bowel sounds per minute in each quadrant
    b. Capillary refill of 5 seconds in a 41-year-old male patient
    c. Respiratory rate of 24 per minute
    d. Systolic pressure of 86 mm Hg
    e. Diastolic pressure of 62 mm Hg

54. You know that it is important to foster rapport and communication with all of your patients. Which of the following actions and interventions would be helpful to increase the effectiveness of your communication and increase nurse–patient rapport?
    a. Talk most of the time you are with the patient so that he or she does not get nervous.
    b. Smile frequently.
    c. Think of a good nickname you can call the patient to put him or her at ease.
    d. Sit in a chair beside the bed and give the patient at least 5 to 10 minutes of your time.
    e. Smile and be genuine.
    f. Always introduce yourself while you are smiling and explain what you are about to do before you perform an intervention or assessment.
    g. Avoid touching the patient to prevent offending him or her.
    h. Be nonjudgmental even when you do not agree with some aspect of the patient's life situations, experiences, beliefs, or opinions.
    i. Be aware of possible cultural restrictions or influences. Verify them when uncertain.

55. Your instructor has asked you to come to the patient's room to hear a good example of a murmur and a bruit. You know that there are specific instances when you use the bell versus the diaphragm side on your stethoscope and when you use light pressure as opposed to pressing to make a firm seal against the patient's skin. Which of the following correctly describes how to use the bell and diaphragm chest piece of your stethoscope?
    a. Use the flat diaphragm to auscultate lower-pitched sounds.
    b. Use the bell to auscultate lower-pitched sounds.
    c. When using the bell, press firmly to seal it against the skin.
    d. When using the flat diaphragm, press it firmly to seal it against the skin.
    e. Murmurs and bruits are considered high-pitched sounds.
    f. The S1 and S2 are considered high-pitched sounds.

Part 4. Application and Critical Thinking Questions

Write a brief answer to the following questions.

56. During examination of the eyes, you check something known as consensual reflex. How is this done?

_____

_____

_____

57. Percussion of a patient's abdomen and chest provides you with what information about the patient?

_____

_____

_____

58. The acronym CTA stands for what? Which means what?

_____

_____

_____

_____

59. The acronym PMI stands for what? Which means what?

_____

_____

_____

60. Explain the importance of performing an initial shift assessment within the first hour of your shift.

_____

_____

_____

61. What assessments should you make of the lower extremities in an initial shift assessment?

_____

_____

_____

Situation Questions

▶ *Scenario: Question 62 refers to this scenario.*

The female patient in Room 314 is 81 years old and is dehydrated. She was too weak to get out of bed at home for several days and has been an inpatient on bedrest for 3 days. She is weak and has to be repositioned every 2 hours or more often as needed to prevent skin breakdown.

62. Describe the assessments that should be performed in relation to these limited data.

_____

_____

_____

_____

▶ *Scenario: Question 63 refers to this scenario.*

Your 76-year-old male patient has renal insufficiency. He is on fluid restrictions of 1500 mL/24 hours. You need to perform a focused assessment of his renal system before discharging another patient who is also assigned to you.

63. Describe the assessments that you will perform to establish the status of his renal system and ensure that he is not getting into fluid overload problems.

_____

_____

_____

_____

_____

▶ *Scenario: Question 64 refers to this scenario. Refer to Figure 21-1.*

A patient with a head injury responds as follows: Opens eyes to pain stimulus. Withdraws from pain. Makes incomprehensible sounds. BP 180/98, P 55 reg, 1+.

64. Score the patient responses on the Glasgow Coma Scale.

_____

Calculate the patient's total score. _____

Would you consider this patient as having a significant neurological impairment?

_____

Function assessed	Patient's response	Score
Eye response	Opens spontaneously	4
	Opens to verbal command	3
	Opens to pain stimulus	2
	No response	1
Motor response	Reacts to verbal command	6
	Reacts to localized pain	5
	Flexes and withdraws from pain	4
	Positions to decorticate posturing*	3
	Positions to decerebrate posturing†	2
	No response	1
Verbal response	Oriented, converses	5
	Disoriented, converses	4
	Uses inappropriate words	3
	Makes incomprehensible sounds	2
	No response	1

* Arms flexed to chest, hands clenched into fists and rotated internally, feet extended: Indicated problem is at or above the brainstem. Also known as *flexor posturing.*

† Arms extended, hands clenched into fists, wrists flexed, and forearms severely pronated (internally rotated): Indicates the problem is at the level of the midbrain or pons and is the more ominous of the two postures. Also known as *extension posturing.* The total points possible ranges from 3 to 15. The highest possible score of 15 indicates that the patient has full level of consciousness (LOC); is awake, alert, and oriented; and follows simple commands. The lower the score, the higher the degree of neurological impairment.

Figure 21.1 Glasgow Coma Scale. (Reprinted from Teasdale G, Jennett B. Assessment of coma and impaired consciousness. A practical scale. *Lancet* 1974;2:81–84.)

Documentation Exercise

Use these initial shift assessment findings for Questions 65 through 68. Record your answers in the forms section at the end of this chapter.

▶ *Scenario:*

Nathan Whitehorse is a 37-year-old Native American male. Today is April 14, 2017. Time: 1115. Medical diagnosis: Newly diagnosed this admission with type 1 diabetes (insulin dependent). He also has an infected wound on the left lower leg that is dressed.

His blood pressure is 153/84. His strength of his lower extremities is strong and equal on both sides (dorsal flexion and also plantar flexion). His apical pulse is 70 beats per minute. His radial pulse is 70 beats per minute. There is no jugular vein distention.

His respirations are 19 per minute. His oral temperature is 98.2°F. He is wide awake and talking. His speech is clear and makes sense. His oxygen saturation level is 98 percent. He is oriented to person, place, time, and situation. He has an IV in his left forearm that is infusing 1,000 mL of half-strength normal saline solution. The IV rate is 30 mL/hr and is controlled by an IV pump. His conjunctivae are both pink and moist. Both of his pupils constrict from 5 mm to 3 mm very quickly when a light is shined in each of them. The right pupil also constricts when shining the light in the left eye and vice versa. When he changes his focus from a distant object to a near object, the pupils constrict and vice versa. His mouth, lips, tongue, and gums are pink and moist, and membranes are intact. His heart sounds are distinct. His heart rhythm and respirations are regular. His breath sounds are clear in all the left lobes and the right upper and right middle lobes, but the right lower lobe has fine rales. His hand grips show the right one to be significantly stronger than the left. He states it is because of a small stroke he suffered 5 years ago. The capillary refill in nailbeds of both hands is brisk. The capillary refill in both feet is sluggish at 5 seconds. The leg wound is 4 inches by 3 inches and 4 mm deep. The base of the wound is pale with only traces of pink. No signs of granulation tissue are noted. There is minimal thin greenish drainage in wound and approximately 2.5-inch diameter dried on the dressing. Edges of wound are red. The patient follows simple commands. He states that he is having a mild discomfort in the wound and surrounding area: a dull, aching pain that is constant, at a 4 on a pain scale of 0 to 10. Denies need for pain medication. He voided 1 hour ago according to the patient and had his last bowel movement last night. States he does not have any other discomforts. His skin is olive, warm, and dry all over except for both feet, which are cool without a color change. His mucous membranes and nailbeds of four extremities are pink. His dorsalis pedal pulse is weak in the left foot and strong in the right foot. He acknowledges that he understands why he needs to drink at least 1500 mL of fluid on this shift and says he is not having any difficulty accomplishing this. His abdomen is flat and feels soft when palpated. He denies any discomfort there. His bowel sounds are hypoactive in the left lower quadrant and active in the other three quadrants. His IV site dressing is intact and there is no redness or edema noted at the site. His pupils are 5 mm in size. He is lying supine and the bed is in low position.

65. Use the nurse's note form (Figure 21-2) to document this faux initial shift assessment in narrative format. Be certain to use correct medical terminology and document it in the correct head-to-toe sequence. Attempt to be succinct. Include your correct signature and credentials.

66. Document the same faux assessment on the patient flow sheet (Figure 21-3).

67. Note the vital signs taken during the assessment in the bottom rows of the graphic sheet, in the "Frequent vs. Monitoring/Reason" area. (Figure 21-4).

68. Document the components of the faux assessment that are part of a neurological examination on the neurological evaluation form (Figure 21-5).

Patient _____		
ID# _____ RM _____		
BD _____-_____-_____		
Admit _____-_____-_____		
Physician _____		

Mission Regional Hospital

Date	Time	Nurse's Notes

Figure 21.2 Nurse's note.

PATIENT FLOW SHEET

(PT STAMP)

	Date:	0700	0800	0900	1000	1100	1200	1300	1400	1500	1600	1700	1800	1900	2000	2100	2200	2300	2400	0100	0200	0300	0400	0500	0600
Care Given	Doctor's visit																								
	Activity																								
	Vital signs																								
	AM care																								
	Turn R-right L-left S-supine P-prone																								
	Dressing wound care																								
	IV therapy																								
	% of diet																								
Skin	Skin intact																								
	Warm-dry/ color WNL																								
	Comfort measures																								
Neuro/ Sensory	Alert & oriented																								
	Denies pain																								
	Denies anxiety																								
Respiratory	O_2 therapy																								
	Breath sounds clear & regular																								
	TC & DB/IS																								
CV	Pulse regular																								
	Heart tones																								
	Telemetry # ___																								
GI	Abdomen soft																								
	Bowel sounds present																								
	BM																								
Renal	Urine clear																								
	Foley patent																								
M/S	Moves all extremities																								
	Side rails up																								
Safety	Call light in reach																								
	Bed in low position																								
Other	Braden scale																								
	Nurse's initials/ signature																								
	Nurse's initials/ signature														RN assessment										
														Time											

CHARTING LEGEND
√ = Within Normal Limits
X = problem, see NN
→ = no change
p = exception is normal for patient
n/a = not applicable

ACTIVITY KEY (x1 or x2 = NURSES ASSISTING)
BED = bedrest
DAN = dangle
CH = chair
AMB = ambulate
BR = bathroom
TUB = tub

ASL = asleep
BP = bedpan
B/B = bedbath
AST = assist
SHR = shower
BSC = bedside commode

O_2 KEY
NC = nasal cannula
M = mask
NRB = non-rebreather mask

HEART TONES KEY
CL = clear
DIM = diminished

COMFORT MEASURES
EM = eggcrate mattress
HP = heel protectors

WOUND DRESSING KEY
√ = dry and intact
D = dressing ▲
SLC = suture line care
I = irrigation

IV KEY
IP = patent
D = dressing ▲
TU = tubing ▲
HL = hep lock
C = central line

Figure 21.3 Patient flow sheet.

GRAPHIC CHART

(PT STAMP)

Hour →		07	11	15	19	23	03	07	11	15	19	23	03	07	11	15	19	23	03	07	11	15	19	23	03

Date: / Date: / Date: / Date:

Temperature: 106° 105° 104° 103° 102° 101° 100° 99° 98.6° 98.5° 98° 97° 96°

Pulse: 150 140 130 120 110 100 90 80 70 60

Respirations: 50 40 30 20 10

BP →

WT →

Frequent vs Monitoring			Reason			Frequent vs Monitoring			Reason		
Date	Time	Temp	Pulse	Resp	BP	Date	Time	Temp	Pulse	Resp	BP

Figure 21.4 Graphic sheet.

NEUROLOGICAL EVALUATION SHEET

2	3	4	5	6	7	8	9
•	•	•	●	●	●	●	●

(PT STAMP)

	0000	0200	0400	0600	0800	1000	1200	1400	1600	1800	2000	2200

Pupil size:
See above

	R	L	R	L	R	L	R	L	R	L	R	L	R	L	R	L	R	L	R	L	R	L	R	L

Pupil reactions:

Brisk	=	3
Slow	=	2
Fixed	=	1

	R	L	R	L	R	L	R	L	R	L	R	L	R	L	R	L	R	L	R	L	R	L	R	L

Motor response:

Obeys commands	=	6
Localizes, defends from pain	=	5
Withdraws from pain	=	4
Abnormal flexion (decorticate)	=	3
Extension response (decebrate)	=	2
Flaccid	=	1

	R	L	R	L	R	L	R	L	R	L	R	L	R	L	R	L	R	L	R	L	R	L	R	L

Eye opening:

Spontaneous	=	4
To speech	=	3
To pain	=	2
None	=	1

Verbal response:

Coherent speech	=	5
Confused conversation	=	4
Inappropriate words	=	3
Incomprehensible sounds	=	2
Mute	=	1

TOTALS →

Nurse signature _____ Date _____

Nurse signature _____ Date _____

Figure 21.5 Neurological evaluation sheet.

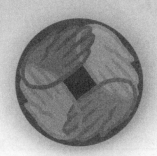

Surgical Asepsis

Name: _____	
Date: _____	
Course: _____	
Instructor: _____	

Part 1. Key Terms Review

Match the following Key Term(s) or italicized words from your text with the correct description.

_____ 1. Disinfection

_____ 2. Boiling

_____ 3. Chemical disinfection

_____ 4. Sterilization

_____ 5. Ionizing radiation

_____ 6. Gaseous disinfection

_____ 7. Autoclaving

a. Sterilization method using steam under pressure

b. Use of steam under pressure, gas, or radiation to kill all pathogens and their spores

c. A method of killing pathogens on sutures, some plastics, and biological material that cannot be boiled or autoclaved

d. A method used to prevent contamination during procedures that involve entering body cavities

e. A method used to kill pathogens on supplies and equipment that are heat sensitive and must remain dry

f. Cleaned with solutions to kill pathogens

g. Used to kill pathogens on equipment and supplies that cannot be heated

h. A method of killing non–spore-forming organisms on instruments and supplies by boiling in water for 10 minutes

Fill in the blank with the correct Key Term(s) or italicized words from your text.

8. _____

is a method used to prevent contamination during

procedures that involve entering body cavities.

9. Another name for the method described in question 8 is

_____.

10. _____ refers to the potential presence of pathogens on a sterile field or sterile object resulting from contact with an unsterile surface.

11. A _____ is an area that is free from all microorganisms where additional sterile items can be placed until they are ready for use.

12. Being aware of potential or certain contamination of the sterile field or sterile objects and taking appropriate steps to correct the contamination is referred to as developing a _____.

13. A registered nurse who assists in the OR by obtaining needed equipment and supplies is called a

_____.

14. A nurse who assists the physician during surgery is called a _____.

Part 2. Connection Questions

Choose the correct answer(s). In some questions, more than one answer is correct. Select all that apply.

15. You are caring for a patient with multiple injuries from a motor vehicle accident. The physician tells you that she wants to insert a chest tube to drain blood from the chest cavity. You know that this is a sterile procedure done at the bedside and you will be needed to assist. Your primary functions will include:
    a. Opening the sterile supplies and placing them on the bedside table
    b. Obtaining the needed equipment and supplies
    c. Checking expiration dates on sterile supplies
    d. Calling surgery and reserving an operating room in case something goes wrong
    e. Obtaining the correct sizes of sterile gloves for the physician, yourself, and anyone else who will be assisting

16. A patient with nerve damage to her bladder tells you that she inserts a catheter to drain her bladder four times a day, but she uses clean technique at home. She questions why you are using sterile technique while she is in the hospital. How will you respond?
    a. "Because your immune system is that strong, sterile technique will not be needed here in the hospital either."
    b. "There are far more microorganisms in the hospital that could cause you harm than the ones at your home, which your body is used to."
    c. "Because I care for other patients, too, I could infect you with pathogens from one of them."
    d. "We have a policy to only use sterile supplies when we are entering any body cavity, so that is what I will do."

17. Which procedures that require sterile technique might be performed by nurses in the long-term care setting?
    a. Administering a vitamin B_{12} injection
    b. Feeding a resident who is unable to feed himself or herself
    c. Inserting a urinary catheter into the bladder
    d. Caring for an open wound
    e. Performing perineal care

18. When you are assisting a physician during a sterile procedure, he asks for more sterile gauze that you have not yet opened. The physician is wearing sterile gloves and you are not. How will you open the gauze and hand it to him?
    a. Peel open the packaging with the opening toward the physician.
    b. Keep your bare hands covered by the packaging.
    c. Remove the gauze from the package and hand it to the physician.
    d. Put on sterile gloves before opening the sterile gauze package.
    e. Allow the physician to remove the gauze from the packaging.

Write a brief answer to the following questions.

19. List two ways you can ensure that your sterile supplies are truly sterile.

    a. _____

    b. _____

20. What could result if you used supplies that had not been adequately sterilized to enter a patient's bladder?

    _____

    _____

Part 3. Review Questions

Choose the correct answer(s). In some questions, more than one answer is correct. Select all that apply.

21. After assisting with a minor surgery in a dermatologist's office, you are asked to clean up the instruments prior to their sterilization. What actions will you take?
    a. Wash them in soapy water, then rinse with clear water.
    b. Leave hinged instruments open.
    c. Rinse the instruments well with cold or warm water.
    d. Dip each instrument in disinfectant solution.

22. How can you tell if a surgical pack has been sterilized?
    a. The peel pack will be sealed all the way around.
    b. The sterilizer's initials will be written on the pack.
    c. The indicator tape hash marks will appear black.
    d. The indicator tape hash marks will disappear.

23. When you obtain a sterile pack, you notice evidence of strike-through. What will you do?
    a. Do not use the pack and dispose of it according to facility policy.
    b. Dispose of the outer wrap because it has been wet and is considered contaminated.
    c. Strike-through means the pack has passed the expiration date and is no longer sterile.
    d. Use the pack as long as the hash marks on the tape have changed colors.

24. You obtain a package of commercially prepared sterile gauze. To ensure it is sterile prior to opening it, you will:
    a. Check the hash marks on the tape to see the color.
    b. Check the stamped expiration date on the package.
    c. Examine the package for any open or unsealed areas.
    d. Look for the date and initials of the person who sterilized the package.

25. Which are restricted areas in the hospital to help maintain surgical asepsis?
    a. Burn units
    b. Pediatric units
    c. Heart catheterization laboratories
    d. Surgical suites
    e. Delivery rooms
    f. Cardiac care units

26. You are assigned to observe in the cardiac catheterization laboratory. What will you do before leaving the unit to go to lunch?
    a. Change from hospital scrubs back into street clothes.
    b. Cover your scrubs with a laboratory coat or cloth isolation gown.
    c. Wear shoe covers over your shoes and a patient gown over your scrubs.
    d. No special precautions are needed when you leave the unit for lunch.

27. It is important to use sterile technique when you insert tubes and needles because:
    a. It is standard hospital policy and procedure, and you must comply with it.
    b. You may be carrying pathogens from patient to patient using only clean technique.
    c. You are entering body tissues not normally exposed to pathogens.
    d. You are bypassing usual body defenses against infection.

28. Which is true of setting up and adding to a sterile field?
    a. The outer 2-inch margin of the sterile drape is considered unsterile.
    b. If the sterile drape extends below the table surface, the parts below it are considered unsterile.
    c. You may place unsterile items on a sterile field as long as you wear sterile gloves.
    d. You may touch the outer 1 inch of the sterile drape with your bare hand because it is considered unsterile.
    e. A sterile drape with a moisture-proof back is not considered unsterile if it becomes wet.
    f. When pouring sterile liquids into a basin on a sterile field, hold the bottle 12 to 14 inches above the basin.

29. You have put on sterile gloves and want to dispose of the wrapper before you proceed. How will you do this?
    a. Wad up the wrapper into a small ball and toss it toward the trash can without bending over.
    b. Carefully pick up the wrapper in the middle and bend at the waist to ensure that it drops into the trash can.
    c. Use your elbow to nudge the wrapper off of the surface and onto the floor; then you can pick it up later.
    d. Grasp the wrapper in the middle, far away from the unsterile outer margin, and drop it from waist height into the trash can.

Indicate the proper sequence of the steps for the following procedure.

30. When you open a sterile pack to set up or add to a sterile field, you will take the following steps. Number them in the correct order.
    _____ a. Open the remaining side flap.
    _____ b. Open the first side flap.
    _____ c. Open the flap toward you.
    _____ d. Open the flap away from you.

Write an "S" for sterile or a "C" for clean technique to indicate which should be used in the following situations.

_____ 31. Inserting a urinary catheter

_____ 32. Washing the perineal area

_____ 33. Administering an insulin injection

_____ 34. Delivering a baby

_____ 35. Handling needles, syringes, and lancets

_____ 36. Inserting a tube through the nose and into the stomach

_____ 37. Inserting an IV needle into a vein

_____ 38. Caring for a patient with severe burns

39. **On the following diagram, label the parts of the needle and syringe that need to be kept sterile.**

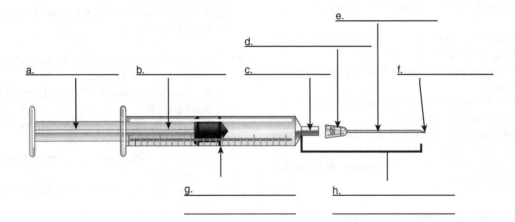

Part 4. Application and Critical Thinking Questions

Write a brief answer to the following questions.

40. Explain the meaning of this principle:
    Sterile + sterile = sterile
    Sterile + unsterile = unsterile
    Unsterile + unsterile = unsterile

    _____

    _____

    _____

41. Describe the boundaries of "Safety Zone" where your sterilely gloved hands must remain.

    _____

    _____

    _____

Situation Questions

▶ *Scenario: Question 42 refers to this scenario.*

You are performing a sterile procedure and are trying to hurry because the patient is scheduled to leave for surgery at any moment. During the procedure you accidentally touch the bedrail with your sterile glove. No one else is in the room, and the patient is not aware of what happened.

42. What will you do? Give the rationale for your actions.

    _____

    _____

    _____

▶ *Scenario: Question 43 refers to this scenario. You will be asked to indicate the sequence of steps for the following procedure.*

You are setting up for a sterile dressing change on a patient who is immunosuppressed. You will need to pour sterile saline into a basin to moisten gauze used to cleanse the wound. You are using a prepackaged dressing change kit that contains all needed supplies including a sterile drape. The container will be used as a sterile basin to hold the saline solution. When you peel back the top of the dressing change tray, you see a sterile drape. No sterile gloves are included in the kit, so you have obtained your correct size to don separately.

43. Number in order the steps you will take to set up your sterile field.

_____ Allow drape to unfold and lay it carefully on the overbed table without touching the sterile surface to anything unsterile.

_____ Don sterile gloves without turning your back on your prepared sterile field.

_____ Open the dressing change tray by peeling back the lid.

_____ Open the sterile saline after checking the expiration date and the date and time if previously opened.

_____ Arrange sterile supplies on a sterile field and place the gauze in the sterile basin of saline.

_____ Carefully dump the contents of the kit onto the sterile field without touching the sterile surface, then set it to the side of the sterile field.

_____ Remove the sterile drape from the kit by handling it only by the edges.

_____ Pour the sterile saline into the empty sterile dressing change tray without splashing.

_____ Recap the sterile saline and avoid touching the inside of the lid.

Documentation Exercise

▶ *Scenario: Questions 44 and 45 refer to this scenario.*

It is January 10, 2017, at 11:30 a.m. You have just assisted Dr. Jacob at the bedside as he inserted a chest tube in Mr. Geoffrey Malik. The patient was medicated before the procedure, as ordered by the physician, and is now resting comfortably. The chest tube immediately started draining 100 mL of dark red fluid. By the end of your shift at 1500, there was 250 mL more of the dark red fluid in the chest tube drainage chamber.

44. Document your assistance of the procedure in the nurse's notes (Figure 22-1) for Mr. Malik.

45. Now document the amount of fluid in the drainage chamber at the end of your shift in the output column of the intake and output record (Figure 22-2). Be sure to total the amount and document the source of the output.

Patient _____		
ID# _____ RM _____		Mission Regional Hospital
BD _____-_____-_____		
Admit _____-_____-_____		
Physician _____		

Date	Time	Nurse's Notes

Figure 22.1 Nurse's note.

Patient _____ Date _____ Shift _____

Intake	Output

Figure 22.2 Intake and output form.

UNIT 4

Clinical Skills and Care

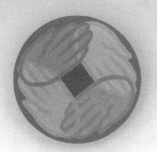

Nutrition

Name:	
Date:	
Course:	
Instructor:	

Part 1. Key Terms Review

Match the following Key Term(s) or italicized words from your text with the correct description.

_____ 1. Absorption

_____ 2. Antioxidants

_____ 3. Body mass index

_____ 4. Digestion

_____ 5. Catabolism

_____ 6. Essential amino acids

_____ 7. Nitrogen balance

_____ 8. Nonessential amino acids

_____ 9. Peristalsis

_____ 10. Complex carbohydrates

_____ 11. Simple carbohydrates

_____ 12. Metabolism

a. Contractions of the gastrointestinal (GI) walls that gently propel the GI contents through the GI tract

b. The process by which nutrients are taken from the end products of digestion into the blood of the capillaries that are located in the villi lining the small intestine

c. Substances that are thought to protect cells from the damage caused by free radicals, thereby promoting good health and preventing disease

d. When the body takes in more nitrogen than it excretes, to use excess nitrogen to build new tissue

e. The process by which body proteins are continuously broken down into amino acids

f. A number calculated from a person's weight and height providing a reliable indicator of body fatness

g. One or two molecules of sugar that are absorbed and burned very quickly; they raise blood glucose level, causing dumping of insulin, which causes the blood glucose level to plummet

h. Amino acids that cannot be made by the body and must be ingested through food

i. Starches and fiber, which take longer to digest than simple sugars; help stabilize blood glucose levels

j. Amino acids made by the body by the breakdown of protein and other excess amino acids

k. The physical and chemical processes in the body that create and use energy

l. The process in which food is broken down in the gastrointestinal (GI) tract, releasing nutrients for the body to use

Part 2. Connection Questions

Choose the correct answer(s). In some questions, more than one answer is correct. Select all that apply.

13. Which two gender and age groups normally require more calories than the others?
    a. 2- to 3-year old male
    b. 17-year-old female
    c. 15-year-old male
    d. 39-year-old female
    e. 63-year-old male

14. It is recommended that adults older than 50 years include food sources or supplements that are fortified with which of the following nutrients?
    a. Crystallized magnesium
    b. Trans vitamin A
    c. Low-density vitamin C
    d. Crystalline form B_{12}

15. It is recommended that women who may become or are pregnant should consume adequate:
    a. Synthetic folic acid daily from fortified foods or supplements
    b. Enhancers of iron absorption, such as vitamin C–rich foods
    c. Food forms of folic acid such as spinach, dried beans, peas, and citrus fruits
    d. Foods high in heme-iron, iron-rich plant foods, or iron-fortified foods

16. Salivary amylase begins to break down:
    a. Proteins
    b. Fat
    c. Simple carbohydrates
    d. Complex carbohydrates

17. The section of the gastrointestinal tract where no digestion takes place is the:
    a. Mouth
    b. Esophagus
    c. Stomach
    d. Small intestine

18. Most absorption of nutrients occurs in the:
    a. Duodenum and jejunum
    b. Stomach
    c. Ileum
    d. Ascending colon

19. For nutrients to be utilized, they must first be absorbed into the bloodstream from the gastrointestinal (GI) tract. This is accomplished by uptake of the nutrients into the:
    a. Arteries providing the GI tract with blood supply
    b. Veins carrying deoxygenated blood away from the GI tract
    c. Capillaries located in the intestinal wall villi
    d. Vessels in the pylorus of the stomach

20. The digestive enzymes needed to digest starches and proteins are released from the:
    a. Liver and gallbladder
    b. Lymphatic system
    c. Pancreas and small intestine
    d. Cecum
    e. Ascending colon

21. Small amounts of electrolytes and nutrients—and most of the water—are absorbed by the:
    a. Stomach
    b. Duodenum
    c. Jejunum
    d. Colon and rectum

22. Nutrients absorbed into the bloodstream from the GI tract travel to the liver via the:
    a. Hepatic artery
    b. Portal vein
    c. Hepatic vein
    d. Lymphatic system

23. What is the minimum amount of water that should be ingested by the average adult in a 24-hour period?
    a. 240 mL
    b. A half liter
    c. 1440 mL
    d. 3 liters
    e. 6 cups

24. Water has several important functions in the body. Which of the following are functions of water?
    a. To help maintain body temperature
    b. To help maintain blood pressure
    c. To dilute the waste products in the blood
    d. To flush toxins from your system
    e. To carry nutrients to the tissue cells

25. Which of the following groups of individuals require the highest level of water intake for optimal health?
    a. Infants
    b. Sedentary adult women
    c. Pregnant women
    d. Elderly men
    e. Nursing mothers

26. Protein is required by the body for:
    a. Producing energy and heat
    b. Building new tissue
    c. Manufacturing hormones and enzymes
    d. Increasing absorption of iron
    e. Forming antibodies
    f. Quick energy

27. Increasing one's fiber intake too much too quickly can have which of the following effects?
    a. Produce excessive gastrointestinal gas
    b. Cause drowsiness
    c. Produce sleeplessness
    d. Increase the appetite
    e. Raise blood pressure

28. The average adult needs how much fiber per day?
    a. 16 ounces
    b. 10 grams
    c. 25–35 grams
    d. 20–25 kcal
    e. 50–100 grams
    f. 6–8 ounces

29. Which of the following vitamins are fat-soluble and can become toxic when stored in the body's fat?
    a. Vitamin A
    b. Vitamin B_{12}
    c. Vitamin K
    d. Vitamin E
    e. Vitamin C
    f. Vitamin D
    g. Vitamins B_1 and B_2

30. Which of the following nutrients cannot be digested and retain their original chemical identities in the body?
    a. Vitamins
    b. Proteins
    c. Minerals
    d. Fats
    e. Simple carbohydrates

31. Kwashiorkor is a type of malnutrition caused by an inadequate dietary intake of:
    a. Vitamin C
    b. Minerals
    c. Healthy fats
    d. Protein

32. Which of the following are correct calorie counts for one gram of each?
    a. Protein 9 kcal, carbohydrates 9 kcal, fat 4 kcal
    b. Protein 9 kcal, carbohydrates 4 kcal, fat 4 kcal
    c. Protein 4 kcal, carbohydrates 4 kcal, fat 9 kcal
    d. Protein 4 kcal, carbohydrates 9 kcal, fat 9 kcal

Part 3. Review Questions

Write a brief answer to the following questions.

33. Identify three factors and describe how they will increase an individual's water needs.

_____

_____

_____

_____

34. Explain what is meant by positive nitrogen balance and how it applies to the rapid growth of childhood and pregnancy.

_____

_____

_____

_____

_____

35. What are LDL and HDL?

_____

_____

_____

_____

_____

36. Provide two examples of pairing incomplete protein food sources that will meet an individual's protein requirements.

_____

_____

_____

_____

_____

Part 4. Application and Critical Thinking Questions

Choose the correct answer(s). In some questions, more than one answer is correct. Select all that apply.

▶ *Scenario: Questions 37 and 38 refer to the following scenario.*

Laboratory results show your patient to be deficient in iron. You are planning a patient teaching session regarding needed dietary changes. You plan to present the material verbally and in a written list of the foods that are considered to be high in iron content.

37. What foods will you teach the patient are high in iron?
    a. Vegetables
    b. Red meats
    c. Fruits
    d. Fish
    e. Poultry
    f. Grains
    g. Beans

38. What nutrient, supplement, or type of food can you teach the patient to use to enhance the absorption of iron?
    a. B vitamins
    b. Vitamin C supplements
    c. Calcium
    d. Yellow vegetables
    e. Citrus fruits

▶ *Scenario: Questions 39 through 42 refer to these two guides and their recommendations.*

You are preparing to teach a patient about basic good nutrition. You plan to use the USDA *Dietary Guidelines for Americans, 2010,* and the ChooseMyPlate.

39. The *Dietary Guidelines for Americans, 2010,* indicates that most U.S. citizens, because of common food consumption patterns, need to do which of the following?
    a. Increase caloric intake and decrease fiber consumption
    b. Increase consumption of dark green and orange vegetables and fruits
    c. Ingest more whole grains and reduce intake of refined grains
    d. Decrease intake of low-fat milk and milk products to prevent osteoporosis

40. ChooseMyPlate recommends which of the following?
    a. Two cups of each of the five food groups at each meal.
    b. Half the plate servings should be fruits and vegetables, and the other half grains and protein foods. Include a serving of dairy.
    c. 1/2 plate protein, 1/6 plate vegetables, 1/6 plate fruits, 1/6 plate grains, tea to drink
    d. Eat more refined grains and simple carbohydrates than protein and fruit.

41. A key recommendation of *Dietary Guidelines for Americans, 2010,* includes reducing sodium intake to 1500 mg/day for which of the following groups of people?
    a. Individuals younger than 50 years
    b. All Native Americans
    c. Individuals with high blood pressure
    d. Individuals with arthritis
    e. Individuals with diabetes
    f. All African Americans

42. The USDA's MyPlate food management system's established recommendations for amounts of food per group are based on which of the following?
    a. Age, gender, and activity
    b. Weight and percentage of body fat
    c. Weight and height
    d. An average of all sizes and ages

Write a brief answer to the following questions.

43. Explain how eating a candy bar and drinking a sugar-loaded cola can drop one's blood glucose level?

_____

_____

_____

_____

44. How can increasing the fiber intake in one's diet lead to a reduced caloric intake?

_____

_____

_____

_____

Documentation Exercise

▶ *Scenario:*

Your patient is Beth Freeland, hospital ID #792283, and she is in Room 312. Her birth date is 6/4/70 and admission date was 8/8/17. Today's date is 8/10/17. It is 1030 and you just completed patient teaching. You verbally presented information regarding Ms. Freeland's specific dietary needs, which is to increase her potassium (K+) and magnesium (Mg+) intake. You told her about a variety of foods that provide K+ and Mg+, including fruits, vegetable, and meats. You knew it would be difficult to remember from memory all the food sources for both nutrients, so you provided her with a written list of foods. She asked several appropriate questions, which you answered. Then she told you, "I will try to really increase how many vegetables and fruits that I eat. I just got out of the habit and have been eating mostly fast foods, burgers and stuff." The foods on the written list that you talked about included OJ, molasses, tomatoes, apricots, trout, cod, tuna, pork, peaches, and prunes for K+, and various nuts, oatmeal, avocado, halibut, peanut butter, and rice for Mg+.

45. On a nurse's note form (Figure 23-1), document this patient teaching session and include evaluation of your effectiveness.

		Mission Regional Hospital
Patient _____		
ID# _____ RM _____		
BD _____-_____-_____		
Admit _____-_____-_____		
Physician _____		

Date	Time	Nurse's Notes

Figure 23.1 Nurse's note.

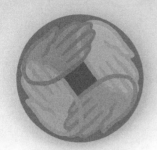

Nutritional Care
and Support

24

Name:	
Date:	
Course:	
Instructor:	

Part 1. Key Terms Review

Match the following Key Term(s) or italicized words from your text with the correct description.

_____ 1. Anaphylaxis

_____ 2. Anorexia nervosa

_____ 3. Bolus feedings

_____ 4. Bulimia nervosa

_____ 5. Enteral nutrition

_____ 6. Parenteral nutrition

_____ 7. PEG tube

_____ 8. Dysphagia

_____ 9. Gastric decompression

_____ 10. NPO

a. Binge eating followed by vomiting or purging

b. Difficulty swallowing; choking

c. Process of reducing the pressure within the stomach by emptying it of its contents

d. A life-threatening allergic reaction; involves swelling of the upper respiratory tract, which can result in occlusion of the airway

e. Relentless self-starvation in an effort to reduce the body weight below normal

f. Intermittent instillation of formula into the PEG tube

g. Nutrients administered directly into the bloodstream via a central venous catheter, bypassing the GI tract

h. Feeding apparatus that goes through the skin into the stomach

i. Restricted intake; nothing by mouth

j. Delivery of tube feedings via the gastrointestinal tract; usually replaces all oral intake

Fill in the blank with the correct Key Term(s) or italicized words from your text.

11. A diet that does not include solid foods and consists entirely of liquids through which you can see is what type of diet? _____

12. An adverse reaction to a food that does not involve the immune system, can stem from the body's lack of digestive enzymes or an inability to use these enzymes, and generally is gastrointestinal in nature is called _____.

13. Food that has been blended to a consistency thicker than a liquid but still can be swallowed easily is found on what type of diet? _____

14. The test that measures the amount of glucose present in the blood over a period of 2 to 3 months, giving a better overall picture of glycemic control, is known as _____.

15. A tube that is inserted through the nose, down the esophagus, and into the stomach is known as an _____.

16. The diet that includes all clear liquids and those fluids that are too opaque to see through is known as _____.

17. Nutrition that is administered through a central venous catheter placed in a larger central vein is known as _____.

18. Nutrition administered through a peripheral intravenous central catheter inserted into a smaller peripheral vein is known as _____.

19. The amount of formula remaining in the stomach from the previous tube feeding is known as _____ and must be assessed prior to every instillation of liquid.

Part 2. Connection Questions

Choose the correct answer(s). In some questions, more than one answer is correct. Select all that apply.

20. Because it is important for patient healing and recovery to ensure optimal nutritional intake, it is helpful for you to provide patients with a pleasant and comfortable environment for mealtimes. Which of the following actions should you perform?
    a. Provide the patient with a warm, wet washcloth to wash his or her face and hands.
    b. Wear lightly fragranced cologne or aftershave to make the patient's room smell nice when you deliver the meal tray.
    c. Remove urinal, toilet paper, hairbrush, or anything you would not want on your home kitchen table during mealtime from the over-the-bed table where the meal tray will be placed.
    d. Use a damp cloth to wipe off the over-the-bed table surface before placing a meal tray on it.
    e. Have the patient lie supine for meals.
    f. Place the over-the-bed table and meal tray in front of the patient, whether the patient is in the bed or sitting in a chair.

21. How much fluid should the average adult take in each day?
    a. 500 mL or less
    b. 500 to 1000 mL
    c. 1000 to 1500 mL
    d. 1500 to 2500 mL
    e. 2500 to 3500 mL

22. When a patient's immune system reacts to a food protein or other large molecule that has been eaten, this is known as:
    a. A food allergy
    b. A food intolerance
    c. An eating disorder
    d. Dysphagia

23. Symptoms of food intolerance generally include which of the following?
    a. Flatulence
    b. Wheezing
    c. Hives
    d. Swelling of the airway

24. Diets modified by consistency include all of the following except:
   a. Clear liquid diet
   b. Mechanical soft diet
   c. Low-sodium diet
   d. Pureed diet

25. The primary component(s) supplied by a clear liquid diet is(are) which of the following?
   a. Protein
   b. Calories
   c. Vitamins
   d. Fluid
   e. Fats

26. A mechanical soft diet sometimes is ordered for patients with severe weakness and fatigue. Which of the following nutrients is not abundant in this diet?
   a. Protein
   b. Fiber
   c. Fat
   d. Vitamins

27. Mike Gibson, a 67-year-old male patient, has been on a liquid diet for several days and is expected to remain on it for at least another week or two. What nutrient(s) will the dietician most likely recommend be added to Mr. Gibson's diet?
   a. Extra water
   b. Fiber
   c. Protein
   d. Calories

28. José Rivera is hospitalized with congestive heart failure and is retaining fluids. Which of the following therapeutic diets is most apt to be ordered for José?
   a. Low-sodium diet
   b. High protein diet
   c. Clear liquid diet
   d. Calorie-restricted diet

29. Haddad Akbar has a severe large decubitus that the hospital staff is working to heal. What type of diet would best meet the needs of this patient?
   a. Full liquid diet
   b. Protein-restricted diet
   c. Renal diet
   d. Diabetic diet
   e. High-calorie, high-protein diet

30. Becca Brennemann, a 16-year-old female, is 5'6" and weighs 97 pounds. She has been exhibiting the following signs and symptoms over the past few months: diarrhea, dehydration, and frequent sore throats. Which of the following is most likely to be the source of her health problems?
   a. Bulimia nervosa
   b. Multiple food allergies
   c. Anorexia nervosa
   d. Lactose intolerance

31. A patient has taken an H_2 blocker for her ulcer disease for several years. She is careful to maintain a nutritionally balanced diet, but a blood test shows that she is deficient in at least one major nutrient. H_2 blockers are known to sometimes interfere with absorption of which nutrient(s)?
   a. Vitamin B_{12}
   b. Vitamin C
   c. Iron
   d. Magnesium
   e. Folate

32. The largest portion of nutrients is absorbed into the bloodstream from the:
   a. Stomach
   b. Small intestine
   c. Liver
   d. Large intestine

33. Most water absorption occurs in the:
   a. Stomach
   b. Small intestine
   c. Liver
   d. Large intestine

34. The purpose of the blue pigtail of a double-lumen nasogastric (NG) tube is to:
   a. Allow instillation of fluids into the stomach while leaving the other lumen plugged.
   b. Instill formula if the primary lumen clogs.
   c. Serve as an air vent.
   d. Prevent the tube from adhering to the stomach wall during decompression.

35. Which action is considered the most reliable for checking tube placement to confirm the correct initial placement of the NG tube after insertion?
   a. Aspirate contents.
   b. Measure the pH of aspirate.
   c. Take an x-ray.
   d. Measure the length of the tube that extends from the nares.

Part 3. Review Questions

Choose the correct answer(s). In some questions, more than one answer is correct. Select all that apply.

36. Which of the following actions should be performed prior to beginning an intermittent tube feeding?
    a. Raise the head of the bed 30 to 45 degrees.
    b. Keep the formula refrigerated until the exact time to instill.
    c. Verify tube placement.
    d. Assess residual gastric volume.

37. The most common foods allergies include some of the following. Which one(s) should not be included?
    a. Peanuts
    b. Bananas
    c. Wheat
    d. Eggs
    e. Dairy products

Write a brief answer to the following questions.

39. What does it mean to decompress the stomach?

_____

_____

_____

_____

_____

_____

40. Explain the difference between a Salem sump tube and a Levine tube.

_____

_____

_____

_____

_____

_____

38. How often during continuous tube feedings should tube placement and residual gastric volume be assessed?
    a. Each time the bag is refilled with formula
    b. Once per shift
    c. Every 4 hours
    d. Every 2 hours

41. How do you prevent air from entering the tube during instillation of a bolus tube feeding by gravity?

_____

_____

_____

_____

_____

42. You are caring for a patient with a nasogastric (NG) tube to low intermittent suction. What are your nursing responsibilities for NG tube care?

_____

_____

_____

_____

_____

_____

_____

_____

_____

_____

_____

_____

Part 4. Application and Critical Thinking Questions

Choose the correct answer(s). In some questions, more than one answer is correct. Select all that apply.

43. Jade Hammond, a 17-year-old female patient, is having an allergic reaction after eating a peanut butter sandwich. You know to be concerned when you observe which of the following signs or symptoms indicative of an anaphylactic reaction?
    a. Rash and itching
    b. Dyspnea
    c. Diarrhea
    d. Bloating

Situation Questions

◗ *Scenario: Questions 44 through 46 refer to this scenario.*

You have been assigned to care for Nancy Counts, who has a small bowel obstruction and is NPO. She has an NG tube to low intermittent suction that has been draining over 600 mL/12-hour shift.

44. When you are prepared to assess Ms. Count's bowel sounds, what should you do first?
    a. Place her in a high-Fowler's position.
    b. Palpate the abdomen for tenderness.
    c. Clamp the NG tube.
    d. Aspirate NG tube contents using a syringe.

45. Ms. Counts later complains that she is feeling nauseated and thinks her stomach is bloated. You are suspicious that which problem has occurred?
    a. The NG tube has clogged.
    b. The suction device has stopped.
    c. The small bowel obstruction has been relieved.
    d. She has been sneaking drinks of fluid.

46. Which of the following assessments should you make every 2 to 4 hours?
    a. Determine the patency of the tube.
    b. Observe the color, amount, and clarity of the aspirate.
    c. Auscultate bowel sounds.
    d. Observe shape of abdomen.
    e. Palpate whether it is firm or soft.

47. Which of the following types of supplemental nutrition can be administered through a smaller peripheral vein?
    a. PPN
    b. TPN
    c. Only mildly hypertonic or isotonic fluids
    d. Hypertonic fluids

48. While caring for a patient receiving total parenteral nutrition, you know to monitor laboratory test results for nutritional status. Which of the following tests provide you with information about the patient's nutritional status?
    a. Electrolytes
    b. WBC
    c. Prealbumin
    d. Total protein
    e. Glucose level

49. When assisting a patient who has been blind for a long time with a meal, it is important to remember:
    a. To approach the situation judiciously and compassionately
    b. That the patient may still be sensitive about the loss of independence
    c. That you should ask the patient if you can help feed him or her
    d. Someone who has been blind for a long time will not want your assistance to eat

50. When evaluating the patient's intake of a meal, be certain to assess for which of the following?
    a. The percentage of food eaten
    b. The patient's ability to tolerate the diet, monitoring for abdominal distention, cramping, nausea, or vomiting
    c. Signs of difficulty swallowing: gagging, choking, or excessive coughing
    d. The level of independence and amount of assistance required
    e. The amount of oral fluid intake: measured, not estimated

Write a brief answer to the following questions.

51. How can you encourage optimal intake while assisting a patient with a meal?

_____

_____

_____

_____

_____

_____

52. What supplies should you gather prior to inserting an NG tube and attaching low, intermittent suction?

_____

_____

_____

_____

_____

53. What tips can you provide the patient to ease the insertion of an NG tube?

_____

_____

_____

_____

_____

_____

_____

_____

_____

_____

54. Why would it be unsafe to use a petrolatum product, such as Vaseline, for lubrication of an NG tube?

_____

_____

_____

_____

_____

_____

55. What are the various methods used to verify tube placement prior to instillation of anything into the NG tube?

_____

_____

_____

_____

_____

_____

Documentation Exercise

▶ *Scenario: Question 56 refers to this scenario.*

Your shift supervisor assigns you to Kay Hudson, a 47-year-old female patient who was admitted this morning for abdominal pain and intermittent nausea of 2 days' duration. She was dehydrated and the physician ordered an IV of 1/2 NS to infuse at 100 mL/hr. She began vomiting this afternoon and complaining of increasing abdominal pain; she received an injection of pain medication just before the end of the shift. She had not voided yet when the off-going nurse gave you a report. The physician has voiced concerns that she may be obstructing her small bowel and wants an update on her status. You also have a second patient, Margaret Gruntmeir, an 81-year-old female who is confused and combative, and needs to have an IV initiated so that she can be given some extra fluids. She has very poor veins and you know that it may keep you tied up for a while gathering your supplies, finding an acceptable vein, and performing the IV initiation, all the while trying to keep the patient calm and still. Your priority is to perform a focused GI assessment along with any other pertinent assessments on Kay Hudson so you can notify the physician. Then you can focus on the IV initiation for Margaret Gruntmeir.

56. Document using a nurse's note form (Figure 24-1) a narrative assessment of a focused GI assessment and any other assessments that you consider pertinent to perform on Ms. Hudson before you can proceed with admitting Ms. Gruntmeir.

57. You suspect a patient is experiencing hypoglycemia. What are the signs and symptoms for which you should assess? List at least six. If you find several of these signs and symptoms, what should be your first intervention?

_____

_____

_____

_____

_____

_____

58. A patient's finger stick blood sugar (FSBS) is 45 mg/dL. The patient is conscious, but
    it is more than 2 hours until the next meal. What interventions should you perform?

_____

_____

_____

_____

_____

_____

		Patient _____	Mission Regional Hospital

Patient _____
ID# _____ RM _____
BD _____-_____-_____
Admit _____-_____-_____
Physician _____

Mission Regional Hospital

Date	Time	Nurse's Notes

Figure 24.1 Nurse's note.

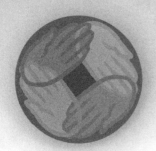

Diagnostic Tests

Name:	_____
Date:	_____
Course:	_____
Instructor:	_____

Part 1. Key Terms Review

Match the following Key Term(s) or italicized words from your text with the correct description.

_____ 1. CBC

_____ 2. WBC

_____ 3. PLT

_____ 4. Hgb

_____ 5. Hct

_____ 6. H&H

_____ 7. CXR

a. Measures the amount of iron pigment in the blood

b. Measures the percentage of red blood cells compared with the whole volume of blood

c. A radiographic picture of the upper torso

d. Measures the number of leukocytes, platelets, and erythrocytes; the hemoglobin; and hematocrit in the blood

e. Measures the number of infection-fighting leukocytes in the blood

f. Measures the protein level in the blood

g. Measures the number of thrombocytes that aid in the blood-clotting process to prevent hemorrhage

h. Measures the amount of iron pigment and the percentage of red blood cells compared with the whole volume of blood

Match the following Key Term(s) or italicized words from your text with the correct description.

_____ 8. Thrombocytopenia

_____ 9. Leukocytosis

_____10. Differential

_____11. Left shift

_____12. Leukopenia

a. An elevation of immature neutrophils called *bands,* which generally indicates bacterial infection

b. An elevation of the complete white blood cell count

c. The percentage of the total white blood cell count
that is made up by each of the five types of white
blood cells

d. A decreased level of platelets

e. An increased level of thrombocytes

f. A low white blood cell count

Fill in the blank with the correct Key Term(s) or italicized words from your text.

13. Basophils are a type of _____ blood cells.

14. Leukocytes are what type of blood cell?

_____

15. Eosinophils are a type of _____ blood cell.

16. Thrombocytes are blood cells whose primary function

is _____.

17. Monocytes are what kind of blood cells?

_____

18. Erythrocytes are _____ blood cells.

19. Lymphocytes are _____ blood cells.

20. What type of blood cell are neutrophils?

_____

Match the acronym with the name of the corresponding test.

_____ 21. CBC

_____ 22. WBC

_____ 23. PLT

_____ 24. Hgb

_____ 25. Hct

_____ 26. H&H

_____ 27. CXR

a. Hemoglobin and hematocrit

b. Hematocrit

c. Chest x-ray

d. Complete blood cell count

e. Hemoglobin

f. White blood cell count

g. Platelet

Part 2. Connection Questions

Choose the correct answer(s). In some questions, more than one answer is correct. Select all that apply.

28. You are responsible for providing patient teaching for
scheduled diagnostic tests. Which of the following
should be included?

a. The cost of the test

b. Purpose of the test

c. The risks involved with the test

d. Any required preparation for the test

e. Chronic pain

29. Which of the following would be helpful during patient
teaching about diagnostic tests?

a. Use correct medical acronyms and terminology to
increase the patient's confidence in your knowledge
about the diagnostic test.

b. Avoid using pamphlets or brochures with pictures of
the diagnostic equipment because they tend to make
the test equipment larger than they really are, which
can increase the patient's anxiety.

c. Assess whether the patient prefers to discuss the test
verbally or to read about it before discussing it.

d. Use terminology that the patient will understand.

30. Preparations for various diagnostic tests commonly include which of the following?
    a. Making the patient NPO
    b. Obtaining written consent
    c. Administering a laxative
    d. Administering medication

31. The preparation for a colonoscopy includes which of the following?
    a. Ingestion of a clear liquid diet 1 to 2 hours before the test
    b. Restriction from ingesting anything green for 24 hours before the examination
    c. Administration of laxatives
    d. Insertion of a Foley catheter

32. After the age of 50 years, it is recommended that a colonoscopy should be performed how often?
    a. Annually
    b. Every other year
    c. Every 5 to 10 years
    d. Once, unless a problem is noted

33. Chest x-rays are useful to detect what?
    a. Atelectasis
    b. The position and size of the heart
    c. Any congestion that is present
    d. The tidal lung volume

34. Prior to an MRI, it is important to assess for:
    a. Claustrophobia
    b. Problems evidenced by the patient's last ECG
    c. Impairment of hearing acuity
    d. Any metal that is within the body

35. What situations or conditions may result in elevated basophil level?
    a. Anaphylactic reactions
    b. Infection
    c. Parasite infestation
    d. Anemia

36. Which of the following blood tests, when below normal, reduces the blood's oxygen-carrying capacity?
    a. Platelet level
    b. White blood cell count
    c. Hemoglobin level
    d. Thrombocyte count

37. A patient was admitted to rule out renal failure. Which of the following diagnostic tests would be most helpful in this situation?
    a. Bilirubin level
    b. UA
    c. Troponin level
    d. GFR

Part 3. Review Questions

Choose the correct answer(s). In some questions, more than one answer is correct. Select all that apply.

38. Which of the following components should not be present in normal urinalysis results?
    a. Glucose
    b. Protein
    c. 0 to 5 WBCs
    d. 20 to 40 RBCs
    e. Ketones
    f. Bilirubin

39. The bilirubin level is used to evaluate the function of the:
    a. Pancreas
    b. Liver
    c. Spleen
    d. Kidneys

40. Before performance of a computed tomography (CT) scan, it is vital to assess which of the following?
    a. Allergy to eggs
    b. Allergy to iodine
    c. Allergy to shellfish
    d. Allergy to gluten

41. Before having CT dye, you should also assess for which of the following?
    a. Wide pulse pressure
    b. Atelectasis
    c. Elevated white blood cell count
    d. Impaired renal function

Part 4. Application and Critical Thinking Questions

Choose the correct answer(s). In some questions, more than one answer is correct. Select all that apply.

42. You are caring for a patient who is scheduled for a paracentesis in the morning. Your patient preparation should include which of the following?
    a. The patient must be NPO for 12 hours prior to the paracentesis.
    b. Tell the patient it will be painless.
    c. Measure the girth of the patient's abdomen.
    d. Assess the patient's weight.

43. The appropriate nursing care for the patient who has just undergone a paracentesis would include which of the following?
    a. Document volume of fluid removed.
    b. Monitor for syncope.
    c. Monitor vital signs.
    d. Keep the patient supine with the head of the bed lower than the foot.

44. The post-test nursing care following a lumbar puncture should include some of the following interventions. Which one(s) would not be included?
    a. Keep patient's bed flat for 8 hours (may turn to lateral position if desired).
    b. Maintain NPO for 4 to 6 hours post-test.
    c. Administer post-test sedative.
    d. Monitor needle insertion site for leakage of spinal fluid.

Write a brief answer to the following questions.

48. A bone marrow aspiration is performed for what purpose?

_____

_____

_____

_____

49. Name two tests that provide data relating to blood flow.

_____

_____

50. What test would evaluate whether a patient has diabetes mellitus?

_____

45. The appropriate test to evaluate whether a patient has kidney stones would be:
    a. A GTT
    b. An IVP
    c. A BE
    d. A chemistry test

46. Which of the following would be categorized as cardiac enzymes?
    a. Troponin
    b. CK-MB
    c. BUN
    d. ALT
    e. AST

47. The diagnostic tests that will produce and record images of tissue and organs, done in sequential slices, include:
    a. CXR
    b. MRI
    c. EGD
    d. CT

51. What test could be done to stage Hodgkin's disease?

_____

_____

Documentation Exercise

52. Determine what should be included in patient teaching in preparation for a barium enema. Document the teaching on a nurse's note form (Figure 25-1), including the effectiveness of the teaching. Be accurate, thorough, and succinct.

		Mission Regional Hospital
Patient _____		
ID# _____ RM _____		
BD _____-_____-_____		
Admit _____-_____-_____		
Physician _____		

Date	Time	Nurse's Notes

Figure 25.1 Nurse's note.

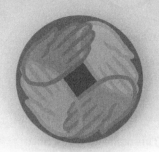

Wound Care

Name: _____	
Date: _____	
Course: _____	
Instructor: _____	

Part 1. Key Terms Review

Match the following Key Term(s) or italicized words from your text with the correct description.

_____ 1. Purulent

_____ 2. Erythema

_____ 3. Ischemia

_____ 4. Necrotic

_____ 5. MRSA

_____ 6. Hemorrhage

_____ 7. Débridement

_____ 8. Eschar

_____ 9. Pressure ulcer

a. Dead tissue
b. Wound drainage containing pus
c. Bleed profusely
d. Redness of skin
e. Resistant strain of *Staphylococcus aureus*
f. Reduced blood flow to tissues
g. Remove by cutting
h. Hard, dry, dead tissue with a leathery appearance
i. Wound resulting from pressure or friction

Fill in the blank with the correct Key Term(s) or italicized words from your text.

10. A patient has an injury on his arm where the skin has been scraped. This injury is a/an _____.

11. New tissue that looks red and semi-transparent that grows to fill in a wound is called _____.

12. Your sister accidentally cut her finger while slicing tomatoes. This injury is a(n) _____.

13. A patient's abdominal wound starts to separate, revealing the inner layers of muscle. This is called wound _____.

14. A _____
    is a channel or tunnel that develops between two cavities
    or between an infected cavity and the surface of the skin.

15. When a patient tries to lift a piano shortly after surgery,
    his abdominal incision separates, and his intestines pro-
    trude through it. This is called a(n) _____.

16. The drainage from a patient's wound is pink. This
    drainage is described as _____.

17. The drainage in a patient's Jackson-Pratt drain is red
    and appears bloody. This drainage is described as

    _____.

18. The drainage on the dressing over a patient's old IV site
    is clear and slightly yellow. This drainage is described

    as _____.

Part 2. Connection Questions

Choose the correct answer(s). In some questions, more than one answer is correct. Select all that apply.

19. During the inflammatory process, the following physio-
    logical responses occur:
    a. Capillaries dilate, causing erythema and increased
       warmth at the site of injury.
    b. Leukocytes are shunted away from the site to fight
       infection.
    c. Leukocytes move into the interstitial space and
       attack microorganisms.
    d. Red blood cells deliver more oxygen and nutrients to
       promote healing.
    e. Fluid in the interstitial spaces prevents redness
       and pain.
    f. Edema causes pressure on nerve endings, resulting
       in discomfort and pain.

20. A patient with an open leg wound has the following
    laboratory results on his chart: WBC 15,350 mm^3 with
    an elevated percentage of neutrophils. What does this
    tell you about the patient's wound?
    a. He most likely no longer has any wound infection.
    b. He most likely has an acute wound infection.
    c. He most likely has a chronic wound infection.
    d. He most likely has a widespread bacterial infection.

21. Which of the following orders would you expect the
    physician to write after receiving laboratory results for
    the patient in question 20?
    a. Bedrest with bathroom privileges
    b. Discharge tomorrow morning
    c. Wound culture and sensitivity
    d. Low-protein diet

22. The nurse realizes that the patient with a shoulder inci-
    sion needs more teaching when the patient says:
    a. "I know the signs of infection and will report them to
       the physician if they occur."
    b. "If my fever goes above 100 degrees, I will notify
       my doctor."
    c. "I know how to change the dressing on my incision
       and have done it three times."
    d. "I will take these antibiotics until the doctor removes
       the staples."

23. An elderly patient who lives alone and has a vascular
    stasis ulcer on his right leg is most at risk for infection
    because he:
    a. May not see well enough to notice changes in the
       wound that indicate infection
    b. Is unable to stay off of his leg, which will compro-
       mise circulation to the area
    c. Does not eat healthy meals, causing a lack of granu-
       lation tissue
    d. Lacks the ability to understand the way that antibi-
       otics work

24. You are a nurse, and you are running behind schedule on
    a very busy workday. The UAP offers to change a pa-
    tient's abdominal dressing for you. She is a first-semester
    nursing student. Which is the most appropriate response?
    a. "That would be great. Don't forget to measure the
       open area in the middle of her incision for me."
    b. "I know you have been taught to do this in school, so
       you are not the same as the other UAPs. Go ahead
       and change the dressing."
    c. "Thanks, but could you help Mr. Wu walk in the hall
       instead? That way I can get that dressing changed."
    d. "You know you can't do that as a UAP. I would be in
       big trouble if I let you change that dressing!"

25. Before you go in the room to change the dressing for your assigned patient, who has a stage III pressure ulcer infected with MRSA, your first priorities will be to:
   a. Determine supplies needed for the dressing change.
   b. Obtain appropriate PPE for caring for a patient with MRSA.
   c. Review sterile technique to prevent contaminating the wound.
   d. Review how to assess a stage III pressure ulcer.
   e. Ask the patient how the other nurses have done the dressing change.

26. Your patient with a stage III pressure ulcer infected with MRSA is on contact precautions. You will obtain the following PPE when you enter his room:
   a. Gloves
   b. Gown
   c. Mask
   d. Goggles

Part 3. Review Questions

Choose the correct answer(s). In some questions, more than one answer is correct. Select all that apply.

27. Classify the following wounds as either open or closed:
   A. Contusion _____
   B. Abrasion _____
   C. Laceration _____
   D. Pressure ulcer _____

28. You are caring for a patient with several risk factors for a pressure ulcer. Which would you avoid when caring for this patient?
   a. Pulling the sheets from beneath the patient so she does not have to turn frequently
   b. Turning the patient using a lift sheet to prevent her from sliding on the sheets
   c. Padding the bony prominences to help prevent pressure that could impair circulation
   d. Turning the patient at least every 2 hours to prevent prolonged pressure in one area

29. A colonized wound is one in which:
   a. There is potential for becoming infected.
   b. Infection is present as a result of gross contamination related to trauma.
   c. Infection is present as evidenced by high numbers of microorganisms and either purulent drainage or necrotic tissue.
   d. A high number of microorganisms are present without signs and symptoms of infection.

30. All of the following are found during your assessment of a surgical wound. Which would concern you the most?
   a. Edges of the wound are together except for a 1-cm area at the distal end, which is open approximately 1.5 cm.
   b. All sutures are intact, but one suture is somewhat looser than the other sutures.
   c. The 2-cm margin around the wound is red, warm, and swollen.
   d. The patient complains of increasing pain in the incisional area compared to yesterday.

31. Which of these patients is most at risk for developing a pressure ulcer?
   a. A well-nourished 54-year-old patient who had a left total knee replacement and is up in the chair twice per day.
   b. A 78-year-old with a feeding tube who is nonambulatory and is incontinent of bowels and bladder.
   c. A 66-year-old who had a myocardial infarction (heart attack) yesterday and is not eating well because of nausea.
   d. A 42-year-old with pneumonia who is receiving IV antibiotics and can only get up to go to the bathroom.

32. A patient has a black, hard, leathery scab on his left heel. The stage of this ulcer is:
   a. Deep-tissue injury
   b. Stage II
   c. Stage III
   d. Unstageable

33. If a patient had a stage III pressure ulcer, you would expect to see which of the following on assessment?
   a. Erythema that remains 15 to 30 minutes after the pressure is relieved and does not blanch
   b. Intact serum-filled blisters and broken blisters with shallow, pink or red shiny ulcerations
   c. An open area that reveals damage to the epidermis, dermis, subcutaneous tissue, muscle, fascia, tendon, joint capsule, and bone
   d. An open area that extends through the epidermis, dermis, and subcutaneous tissue with possible undermining and tunneling

34. While assessing the skin of a patient on bedrest, you notice a pale area over the left hip with a small blister in the center. What action will you take?
    a. Massage the area vigorously with lotion to promote circulation.
    b. Notify the physician that a pressure ulcer has developed.
    c. Document your findings and assess again in 2 hours.
    d. Order a special gel-filled mattress for the patient.

35. A patient comes to the clinic where you are working as a nurse. He had surgery 2 months ago and is very concerned. He asks you to feel the scar on his side. You feel a hard ridge beneath the incision scar extending about 1 cm on either side of the scar. Which response is most appropriate?
    a. "This is a normal part of scar healing and strengthening. It will eventually thin out and become less hard."
    b. "This might be a keloid forming, which is an overgrowth of scar tissue. It is not dangerous."
    c. "This is very unusual at this stage of healing. The doctor will need to look at your scar."
    d. "Don't worry. Different people heal at different rates. You must just be a slow healer."

36. When you assess a patient's skin, you will pay special attention to the color, noting:
    a. Excoriation
    b. Erythema
    c. Smoothness
    d. Pallor
    e. Bruising
    f. Jaundice

37. A patient is at risk for wound dehiscence as a result of nutritional issues and medical history. Which interventions should be included in the care plan?
    a. Assist the patient to splint the incision with a pillow when coughing.
    b. Enforce strict bedrest with bathroom privileges only.
    c. Administer stool softeners and antinausea medicine promptly.
    d. Obtain VS every 15 minutes.

38. In what order do wounds heal?
    a. Reconstruction phase, maturation phase, inflammatory phase
    b. Inflammatory phase, maturation phase, reconstruction phase
    c. Prodromal phase, symptoms phase, inflammatory phase, reconstruction phase
    d. Symptoms phase, maturation phase, inflammatory phase, reconstruction phase

39. Which of these factors affect wound healing?
    a. Positive attitude
    b. Chronic illness
    c. Medications
    d. Atmospheric pressure
    e. Diabetes mellitus
    f. Age

40. A patient has had emergency surgery because of a bowel obstruction. The wound becomes infected with *E. coli*. This likely occurred because:
    a. These bacteria are always present on the skin and easily enter a wound if sterile technique is not used.
    b. These bacteria grow in the absence of oxygen, which is the case in the bowel.
    c. These bacteria are present in the bowel, and with emergency surgery there is no time to perform special bowel preparations.
    d. The patient had poor nutritional intake because these bacteria grow in dying tissue.

41. You are calling a physician to report a possible wound infection. What information will you include in your report?
    a. Most recent vital signs
    b. Amount and type of wound drainage
    c. Observed signs of infection
    d. Type and frequency of bowel movements
    e. Patient's rating of his or her pain
    f. Amount of activity the patient has had in the past 24 hours
    g. Laboratory results

Match the following types of wound healing with their examples.

_____42. First intention

_____43. Second intention

_____44. Third intention

a. A traumatic wound first left open to drain, then sutured closed
b. An appendectomy incision sutured closed
c. A pressure ulcer being packed with moist gauze

Label the following figures.

45.

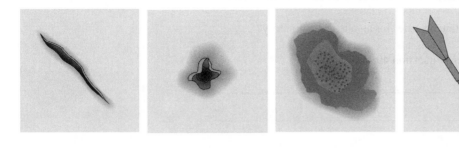 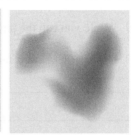

a._____ b._____ c._____ d._____ e._____

_____ _____

Part 4. Application and Critical Thinking Questions

Write a brief answer to the following questions.

◗ *Situation: Questions 46 through 48 refer to this scenario.*

You walk into a patient's room and discover that his abdominal wound has eviscerated.

46. What action will you take first?

_____

_____

_____

_____

47. What will you assess and why?

_____

_____

_____

_____

48. What additional nursing interventions will you perform while waiting for the patient
      to return to the operating room?

_____

_____

_____

_____

▶ *Situation: Questions 49 and 50 refer to this scenario.*

Your patient has a small skin tear. The bleeding has stopped and a scab has formed over it. The area around it is slightly reddened with a very small amount of swelling.

49. Would you call the physician to obtain an order for an anti-inflammatory? _____

50. Explain the reasons for your answer to question 49.

_____

_____

_____

_____

▶ *Situation: Questions 51 through 53 refer to this scenario.*

Your patient is 4 days postop with an abdominal incision. She complains of pain, increasing since yesterday evening. She now rates it an 8 out of 10. She is taking the oral antibiotic azithromycin (Zithromax).

51. What will you assess immediately?

_____

_____

_____

_____

52. What other assessments might you make?

_____

_____

_____

_____

53. There are several abnormal findings in your assessment. What orders would you expect to receive from the physician?

_____

_____

_____

_____

Documentation Exercise

▶ *Scenario:*

You are caring for Chan Nguyen. His identification number is 6487953. His date of birth is 5/5/1939. Today is June 30, 2017. Your patient has a stage III pressure ulcer on his coccyx. It is 2-cm deep at the proximal end and 1-cm deep at the distal end.

At 9:30 a.m. you change the dressing on the wound. Your orders are to apply a wet-to-damp dressing. You use three 4 × 4s and one ABD dressing. A medium amount of pink drainage is seen on the dressing you remove. He complains that it is a bit uncomfortable when you pack the wound, although you had administered pain medication an hour prior to the dressing change. At 10:40 a.m. you return to check on the patient. He looks like he is sleeping. You count his respirations. He is breathing deeply at 14 breaths per minute.

54. Document your dressing change on the nurse's note (Figure 26-1). Review information in the chapter to thoroughly document what you have done and the appearance of the wound.

| Patient _____ |
| ID# _____ RM _____ |
| BD _____-_____-_____ |
| Admit _____-_____-_____ |
| Physician _____ |

Mission Regional Hospital

Date	Time	Nurse's Notes

Figure 26.1 Nurse's note.

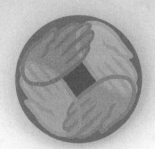

Musculoskeletal Care

Name:
Date:
Course:
Instructor:

Part 1. Key Terms Review

Match the following Key Term(s) or italicized words from your text with the correct description.

_____ 1. Osteoarthritis

_____ 2. External fixator

_____ 3. Sprain

_____ 4. Prosthesis

_____ 5. Fractures

_____ 6. Spica

_____ 7. Amputate

a. An injury to joints that results in damage to muscles and ligaments

b. The type of cast that encases the hips and one or both legs

c. An artificial body part, such as an arm or a leg

d. A disease that causes degeneration and inflammation of the joints over time

e. Surgical removal of a limb as a result of extensive trauma or tissue death

f. The head of the femur and the acetabulum of the pelvis

g. Wires, pins, tongs, or rods used in skeletal traction

h. Breaks in the bone, ranging from a narrow crack to many pieces

Fill in the blank with the correct Key Term(s) or italicized words from your text.

8. A surgery in which damaged articular bone surfaces are removed and replaced with metal and plastic surfaces is called a _____.

9. The term _____ refers to the remaining portion of a limb after an amputation.

10. The health-care team member responsible for assessing musculoskeletal disorders and developing the plan of care to strengthen muscles and restore mobility is

_____.

11. The machine used to gently flex and extend the patient's knee after a total knee replacement is a _____ machine.

12. The type of traction in which the limb is wrapped in an elastic bandage or wrap to which a frame and weights are attached is _____ traction.

13. The type of traction in which external fixators are used is referred to as _____ traction.

Part 2. Connection Questions

Choose the correct answer(s). In some questions, more than one answer is correct. Select all that apply.

14. When you care for a patient prior to surgery, one of your primary concerns is:
    a. Researching the exact surgery that will take place
    b. Ensuring that all preoperative orders are carried out correctly
    c. Showing the family where to wait during the surgery
    d. Explaining the surgical techniques that will be used with the patient

15. When you care for a patient after a joint replacement, a major nursing focus will be:
    a. Teaching the patient about healthy lifestyles
    b. Screening the family for joint diseases
    c. Managing pain and mobility
    d. Preventing complications related to immobility

16. A patient came to the ER complaining of pain in her elbow after a fall. The x-ray shows fractured ulna at the olecranon process. There is also a suspected fracture of the radius. Which diagnostic test would be most helpful in determining a complete diagnosis?
    a. CT scan
    b. MRI
    c. Bone scan
    d. Electromyelogram

17. A 10-year-old has a fractured left leg with no trauma occurring to cause it. The physician diagnoses a pathological fracture, possibly from a bone tumor. What type of diagnostic test would be ordered in this situation?
    a. CT scan
    b. MRI
    c. Bone scan
    d. Electromyelogram

18. The components of the hip joint that form the ball and socket are the:
    a. Pelvis and greater trochanter
    b. Femur and patella
    c. Acetabulum and lesser trochanter
    d. Head of the femur and the acetabulum

19. You are working in a home health setting. Which of the following assessments would cause you to consider asking your supervisor to arrange for a physical therapy referral for your patient?
    a. The patient is ambulating in the home with a walker.
    b. The patient had surgery recently and is holding on to furniture to ambulate.
    c. The patient uses a wheelchair in the home, which has been remodeled to accommodate it.
    d. The patient is able to transfer with the assistance of one person and has a 24-hour caregiver in the home.

20. You are working in a long-term care setting. One of the residents is able to ambulate but sits in a wheelchair each day. What action will you take?
    a. Check the orders for ambulation and be sure that they are followed to promote mobility.
    b. Change the activity order to wheelchair only because the resident prefers to sit rather than ambulate.
    c. Instruct the CNA to do passive range-of-motion exercises because the resident is not ambulating anymore.
    d. Call the doctor and report that the resident is no longer ambulating.

21. Explain the purpose of an abduction pillow.

_____

_____

_____

_____

Part 3. Review Questions

22. Fill in the acronym for the care of a sprain.

    R = _____

    I = _____

    C = _____

    E = _____

Choose the correct answer(s). In some questions, more than one answer is correct. Select all that apply.

23. A common condition that requires a joint replacement is:
    a. A hairline fracture
    b. Osteoarthritis
    c. A comminuted fracture
    d. An amputation

24. The reason(s) that a limb might have to be amputated include:
    a. Severe tissue damage from trauma
    b. Severely decreased blood flow to the limb
    c. Failure of skeletal traction to successfully treat a fracture
    d. Gangrene (death of tissue) in the limb

25. A typical ambulation order by a physician or physical therapist might be:
    a. "Walk patient in hall."
    b. "Ambulate in hall several times."
    c. "Ambulate 24 steps each day."
    d. "Ambulate three times per day, 20 feet (6 meters) each time."

26. Who is responsible for carrying out ambulation orders for patients?
    a. PT only
    b. Nursing assistants only
    c. All nursing staff and PT staff
    d. PT assistants only

27. A type of external fixator composed of metal rings on the outside of the limb with rods and wires attached that penetrate through the skin into the bone is a(n):
    a. External immobilizer
    b. Buck's traction setup
    c. Skin traction setup
    d. Ilizarov frame

28. You are caring for a young child with hip dysplasia who is in a spica cast. An important nursing concern is:
    a. Assessing circulation to the fingers and hands
    b. Moving the patient carefully without using the abductor bar
    c. Keeping the patient's hips elevated above the heart
    d. Aligning the hips each time the patient is turned

29. A patient is admitted with an elevated temperature and complaining of pain under his arm cast. A bad odor is noted coming from the elbow area of the cast. The patient tells you that his arm has been itching a great deal under the cast. What concern do you have?
    a. The patient may have damaged the skin under the cast, causing infection.
    b. The bone is not healing well under the cast, causing the pain.
    c. The skin under the cast is breaking down because of pressure from the cast.
    d. The patient may be developing gangrene (tissue death) under the cast, causing the odor.

30. What patient teaching will you do for the patient described in question 29?
    a. Teach the patient to use a straightened coat hanger padded with gauze to scratch under the cast.
    b. Instruct the patient to use a blow dryer to blow cool air under the cast to relieve itching.
    c. Explain how epidermal cells shed, then build up under the cast, causing itching.
    d. Suggest that the patient blow hot air under the cast with a blow dryer to relieve itching.

31. A patient has a quarter-size amount of drainage on her cast. The next day the amount of drainage has increased to 2 inches (5 cm) in diameter. The nurse would be most concerned about:
    a. Swelling beneath the cast
    b. Neurovascular impairment
    c. Infection under the cast
    d. Placing tape petals over the edges of the cast

32. The purpose of a trapeze bar is to:
    a. Prop the linens off of the patient's legs and feet
    b. Hold the ropes and weights in traction
    c. Provide a hand grip for the patient to use when moving in bed
    d. Provide attachment points for skeletal traction

33. Which would you consider to be significant findings when caring for a patient with skeletal traction?
    a. Redness and swelling at the pin insertion sites
    b. A small amount of serosanguineous drainage at the pin insertion sites
    c. Purulent drainage at the pin insertion sites
    d. Mild discomfort when the patient moves the limb in traction

34. Care of the pin insertion sites includes:
    a. Cleaning the area with hydrogen peroxide or normal saline solution as ordered
    b. Applying antibiotic ointment to the site
    c. Inspecting the site for signs and symptoms of infection
    d. Shaving the hair around the site

35. Which bone components are replaced in a total hip replacement surgery?
    a. The head and neck of the femur and the acetabular cup
    b. The greater trochanter of the femur and the acetabular cup
    c. The ilium and the head of the femur
    d. The distal end of the femur and the head of the tibia

36. A patient who is 3 days post left total hip replacement is sitting in a chair and drops a magazine. How should he or she retrieve it?
    a. Bend laterally at the waist to pick it up.
    b. Bend over with the knees flexed to pick it up.
    c. Call for someone else to pick it up.
    d. Use an extension gripper to pick it up.

37. What are the articular surfaces in a total knee replacement?
    a. A metal tibial component that articulates with the plastic surface of the femoral component
    b. A metal femoral component that articulates with the plastic fibula component
    c. The patella is replaced with plastic or similar substance, or has plastic affixed to the back to provide a smooth articular surface
    d. The patella, tibia, and femur are replaced with plastic or polyethylene components

38. What is the purpose of wrapping a stump after an amputation?
    a. To shape it to fit correctly into the prosthesis
    b. To prevent healing in a squared-off shape
    c. To prevent the incision from breaking open while wearing a prosthesis
    d. To promote healing of the incision

39. You know a patient's crutches fit correctly when:
    a. There is a three-fingerbreadth gap of space between the axillary pad and the patient's axilla.
    b. There is a slight bend in the patient's elbows when standing with the crutches next to his or her feet.
    c. The crutches fit snugly into the axilla when the patient is standing with the crutch tips next to the heels.
    d. There is a 6-inch or larger gap between the patient's axilla and the top of the crutch.

40. A patient states he has fallen twice since using crutches for a foot injury. Which of the following questions might you want to ask him?
    a. "Have you had any physical therapy for balancing exercises?"
    b. "Are you sure your crutch tips are not too slick?"
    c. "Would you show me how you hold your foot when you walk with the crutches?"
    d. "Haven't you ever used crutches before?"

41. What is the advantage of a multipronged cane over a single-tipped cane?
    a. It is easier to adjust to the patient's height.
    b. It can stand by itself rather than having to be leaned against something.
    c. The handle on a multipronged cane is easier to grasp.
    d. It decreases the chances of the cane slipping as the patient leans on it.

42. Which of the following would you include when you teach a patient about using a cane?
    a. Hold the cane on your affected side.
    b. Move the unaffected leg and the cane together, and then move the affected leg.
    c. Lean to the side the cane is on for best support.
    d. All of these are appropriate patient teaching regarding canes.

43. When a walker is correctly fit to a patient, which of the following is true?
    a. The walker will come to the patient's hip.
    b. The top bar of the walker will reach the patient's waist.
    c. The patient's elbows will be bent at a 30-degree angle when his or her hands are on the handles.
    d. The patient's elbows will be bent at a 90-degree angle when the patient is pushing the walker.

44. You are working with a patient whose left leg is weak. You are instructing her on walker use. Which instruction is most appropriate?
   a. "Move your right leg forward with the walker, then move up your left leg."
   b. "Move the walker forward, then move your left leg forward, followed by your right leg."
   c. "Move the walker forward, then move your right leg forward, followed by your left leg."
   d. "Move the walker and your left leg forward at the same time, then move your right leg forward."

45. Label the parts of the hip joint on the following diagram.

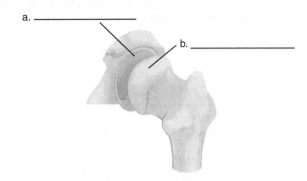

a. _____

b. _____

Write a brief answer to the following questions.

46. When using a walker, where should the patient stand? What is the reason for this?

_____

_____

_____

_____

47. A patient comes into the clinic where you are working for a follow-up visit after breaking her ankle. She has been using crutches for the past 2 weeks and is complaining of pain and tingling in her forearms and hands. What is the most likely cause of these symptoms?

_____

_____

_____

_____

Part 4. Application and Critical Thinking Questions

Choose the correct answer(s). In some questions, more than one answer is correct. Select all that apply.

48. You see the following orders on the Kardex for a patient with a newly applied cast to the right arm. Which order would you question as to its accuracy?
   a. "May petal cast if necessary."
   b. "Support right arm on pillows until the cast is dry."
   c. "Keep the right arm elevated at all times."
   d. "Do neurovascular checks every 4 hrs × 4, then every 8 hrs × 2."

49. You are caring for a patient who had a total knee replacement 2 days ago. She has orders for CPM for 2 hours four times per day at 35 degrees of flexion. Which would concern you the most?
   a. The patient's leg and the CPM machine are in alignment with the rest of the patient's body.
   b. The patient complains of severe pain with each flexion of the knee.
   c. The patient is using relaxation breathing to prevent tensing of the leg muscles while on the CPM machine.
   d. The platform of the CPM machine is centered beneath the patient's knee.

Write a brief answer to the following questions.

50. A patient who has had a total knee replacement asks you to take off the CPM machine after 1 hour, although it is ordered to be on for 2 hours. How will you respond?

_____

_____

_____

_____

51. A patient has a fresh plaster cast applied to the left leg from the thigh to the ankle. How will you prevent complications as the cast dries?

_____

_____

_____

_____

52. A patient has skeletal traction applied to his left lower leg. Why is pin site care critical for this patient?

_____

_____

_____

_____

53. A patient is in skin traction. You notice that when the bed is lowered to its lowest position, the weights are on the floor. Why is this a problem?

_____

_____

_____

_____

Situation Question

▶ *Scenario:*

You are caring for a patient post left hip replacement surgery. You heard in report that the patient is not compliant regarding limiting his hip flexion to no more than 90 degrees. You prepare to teach the patient about flexion restrictions. During your teaching, the patient states, "I never had to be careful how I moved my hip before surgery, and that was when it had bad arthritis in it. Now I have a new replacement, so why would I need to limit how I move it? You say it can dislocate, but it never dislocated before."

54. How will you respond?

_____

_____

_____

_____

_____

Documentation Exercise

You are caring for a patient named Phyllis James, who is 54 years old. She is in Room 157. She has returned to the nursing unit after having surgery to repair a left tibial fracture. She has an immobilizer in place on her lower left leg. You are assigned to do neurovascular checks on this patient. At 4:15 p.m. you do so and you gather the following data:

Her pedal pulses are present in both feet, but the pulse in her right foot is stronger than the pulse in her left foot. She can feel you run a paperclip along the bottom of both her right and her left foot. There is no swelling in her right foot, but her left foot is puffy, with 2+ pitting edema. Her left foot and lower leg are red, but her right foot and leg are pink. She can wiggle her toes freely on her right foot, but the toes on her left foot only move slightly when you ask her to move them. She says she has no pain in her right leg, but her left leg is hurting. She rates the pain at a 5. When you check her capillary refill, you note that both feet are warm to the touch and the toenail beds on both feet refill within 3 seconds.

55. Document your data on the neurovascular checklist (Fig. 27-1).

56. Compare your data with the previous neurovascular check done in the recovery room. Determine if further action is required. If so, document your actions on the nurse's notes (Fig. 27-2).

Neurovascular Checklist

James, Phyllis #245689 Rm. #157 BD 2-10-1963 Admit 3-7-YY	Mission Regional Hospital		
Date _3-9-YY_	**Time** 1420	**Time**	**Time**
Sensation R L	WNL WNL		
Edema R L	None +1		
Skin temperature R L	Warm Warm		
Skin color R L	Pink Red		
Capillary refill R L	Toes—less than 3 seconds Toes—less than 3 seconds		
Movement R L	Wiggles toes freely Wiggles toes freely		
Pulses R L	Present and strong Present and strong		
Pain R L	0 4		

Figure 27.1 Neurovascular checklist.

Patient _____
ID# _____ RM _____
BD _____-_____-_____
Admit _____-_____-_____
Physician _____

Mission Regional Hospital

Date	Time	Nurse's Notes

Figure 27.2 Nurse's note.

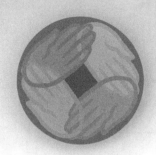

Respiratory Care

Name: _____

Date: _____

Course: _____

Instructor: _____

Part 1. Key Terms Review

Match the following Key Term(s) or italicized words from your text with the correct description.

_____ 1. Cyanosis

_____ 2. Pleural effusion

_____ 3. Dyspnea

_____ 4. Visceral pleura

_____ 5. Endotracheal tube

_____ 6. Incentive spirometer

_____ 7. Hypoxia

_____ 8. Nebulizer

_____ 9. Parietal pleura

_____ 10. Hypoxemia

_____ 11. Hemothorax

a. Oxygen level in the blood below normal range

b. A medication delivery system containing an air compressor and a mouthpiece or mask

c. Blood and drainage in the pleural space

d. Bluish discoloration of the lips, nose, ears, and nailbeds as a result of decreased oxygen

e. The tube inserted into a tracheotomy

f. The portion of the pleural membrane that lines the chest cavity

g. Lack of oxygen taken to the tissues by the blood; a result of hypoxia

h. Fluid in the chest cavity

i. A device used to encourage patients to take frequent deep breaths

j. The portion of the pleural membrane that covers the lungs

k. A firm but flexible tube that is inserted through the nose or mouth to provide air to the lungs

l. Difficulty moving air in and out of the lungs

Fill in the blank with the correct Key Term(s) or italicized words from your text.

12. When air is pulled into the lungs until the pressure in the lungs equals the pressure outside of the body, the result is called _____.

13. Mucus coughed up from the lungs is called _____.

14. When a hole allows air to enter the pleural space, the condition is called a _____.

15. When air is forced out of the lungs as a result of relaxation of the diaphragm and intercostal muscles, it is referred to as _____.

16. A life-threatening situation occurs when air is trapped in the pleural space surrounding the lungs, causing pressure on the lungs, heart, and major blood vessels. This is known as a _____.

17. An incision into the trachea held open with a tube to promote breathing is known as a _____.

18. _____ occurs when there is air in the subcutaneous tissues. It feels like crispy rice cereal being crushed beneath the patient's skin.

19. When a lung collapses, the condition is referred to as _____.

Part 2. Connection Questions

Choose the correct answer(s). In some questions, more than one answer is correct. Select all that apply.

20. When you care for a patient with a tracheostomy, it is important to first research:
    a. The purpose and type of tracheostomy the patient has
    b. How the underlying condition, such as pneumonia, developed
    c. How to correctly suction a tracheostomy
    d. The brand name of the tracheostomy the patient has

21. For the lungs to expand when the chest wall expands, it is important to:
    a. Maintain negative pressure in the pleural space.
    b. Maintain positive pressure in the pleural space.
    c. Prevent excessively large inhalations.
    d. Discourage frequent coughing.

22. Why might a patient with low oxygen saturation misinterpret stimuli?
    a. Low oxygen saturation can result from an impaired breathing pattern, which could be caused by some mental illnesses.
    b. Lack of oxygen to the brain causes the inability to reason and use normal judgment.
    c. Decreased oxygen saturation has an immediate effect on the optic nerves, which are very oxygen sensitive, causing changes in vision.
    d. Low oxygen saturation causes hallucinations and delusions in most people.

23. Arterial blood gases provide information about which values?
    a. Bicarbonate level
    b. Partial pressure of oxygen in the blood
    c. pH of the blood
    d. Carbonic acid level of the blood
    e. Partial pressure of carbon dioxide in the blood
    f. Carbon monoxide level

24. Which of the following aspects of obtaining an arterial blood gas sample are different than obtaining a venous blood sample?
    a. The syringe has a small amount of heparin added to prevent clotting.
    b. The sample is taken from an artery, not from a vein.
    c. After obtaining the sample, the needle is inserted into a cork to prevent air from entering the syringe.
    d. The blood is transported to the laboratory for testing.
    e. The syringe is placed on ice after the sample is drawn.

25. How will you know if your patient teaching about using the incentive spirometer was effective?
    a. The patient will blow forcefully into the spirometer 10 times each hour.
    b. The patient will verbalize that the spirometer will help prevent blood clots in his or her lungs.
    c. The patient will change the settings on the spirometer to a lower number each day.
    d. The patient will demonstrate the correct use of the spirometer and correctly answer questions about its purpose.

26. How can you evaluate the effectiveness of suctioning a patient's tracheostomy?
    a. Ask the patient if he or she can breathe more easily after suctioning.
    b. Auscultate the patient's lungs for a decrease in clear breath sounds.
    c. Measure the amount of fluid suctioned out of the tracheostomy. If it is more than 50 mL, the suctioning was effective.
    d. Listen to see if the patient is breathing easily without rattling or gurgling.

Part 3. Review Questions

27. Number in order the structures that air passes through as it enters the respiratory system.
    _____ Trachea
    _____ Bronchioles
    _____ Nostrils
    _____ Right or left bronchus
    _____ Pharynx
    _____ Alveoli

Choose the correct answer(s). In some questions, more than one answer is correct. Select all that apply.

28. Which description is most accurate regarding the mechanics of breathing?
    a. Breathing is voluntary because people are able to hold their breath at will.
    b. Breathing is involuntary and occurs because of the movement of the diaphragm and intercostal muscles.
    c. When the diaphragm contracts, it moves upward and the intercostal muscles move the ribs up and out, causing expiration.
    d. In the alveoli, oxygen leaves the alveoli and moves into the blood in the capillaries as a result of osmosis.

29. Contraction of the diaphragm is initiated by the:
    a. Cerebellum sending chemicals to the chemoreceptors
    b. Changes in pH of the blood, detected by the carotid arteries
    c. Changes in position of the ribs as a result of the contraction of the intercostal muscles
    d. Medulla sending impulses to the phrenic nerve

30. You have been asked to explain internal and external respirations to another student. Which explanation(s) will you use?
    a. External respiration occurs inside the body, and internal respiration occurs outside the body.
    b. Internal respiration occurs when oxygen and carbon dioxide are exchanged between the bloodstream and the body cells.
    c. Internal respiration occurs as a result of diffusion of oxygen from the alveoli to the blood; external respiration occurs as a result of osmosis of oxygen from the blood into the lungs.
    d. External respiration occurs when oxygen and carbon dioxide are exchanged between the alveoli and the lung capillaries.

31. Which of the following signs and symptoms would indicate that your patient is *beginning* to become hypoxic?
    a. Bluish coloration to lips and nailbeds
    b. Becomes irritated when you try to help him turn in bed
    c. Respiratory rate change from 16 to 24
    d. Heart rate change from 72 to 60
    e. Thought he was at a hotel, but then knew he was at the hospital this morning
    f. Complaints of pain above his eyes

32. Your patient has recently woken from a nap. She thinks it is morning, although it is 3 o'clock in the afternoon. She also thinks you are her daughter-in-law. When you take her vital signs, her pulse is 56 and irregular, her respiratory rate is 28, and she is having difficulty taking a deep breath. Her earlier vital signs were T 99.2, P 66, R 18, and BP 134/76. What concerns do you have about this patient?
    a. She may be having a CVA because she is confused.
    b. She may have a pulmonary embolus because she is having difficulty taking a deep breath.
    c. She may be hypoxic because her vital signs have changed and so has her orientation.
    d. She may be having a heart attack because her heart rate has dropped 10 beats per minute and become irregular.

33. Your patient has been diagnosed with *Pseudomonas* pneumonia and has thick secretions in his lungs. You are most concerned about:
    a. Spread of the infection from his lungs to other parts of his body
    b. Transmitting the infection to other patients on the nursing unit
    c. Impaired oxygenation as a result of thick secretions in his alveoli
    d. Performing the Heimlich maneuver to clear his airway

34. You are caring for a patient who is severely anemic and has atelectasis of the left lung. These conditions can easily lead to:
    a. Hypoxia and hypoxemia
    b. Infection and sepsis
    c. Asthma attack and stroke
    d. Hallucinations and delusions

35. As you assess your patient with dark skin tone, you notice that the color of her skin is ashen. What will you do next?
    a. Increase the temperature of the room because the patient is most likely too cold.
    b. Assess the patient's mucous membranes, palms, and soles of the feet for evidence of cyanosis.
    c. Ask the patient's family if this color is normal for her.
    d. Take a set of vital signs, paying special attention to the blood pressure.

36. How can you assess a patient for exertional dyspnea?
    a. Ask the patient if he feels short of breath during meals.
    b. Count the patient's respirations at rest and note the number of breaths higher than 22 per minute.
    c. Compare the patient's respiratory rate at rest with the respiratory rate when the patient ambulates for even a short distance.
    d. Assess oxygen saturation during sleeping and during talking, and compare the difference.

37. When making an assessment on a young child, you note retractions around the ribs and the sternum. Which action will you take first?
    a. Notify the physician immediately.
    b. Obtain a sputum specimen via suction.
    c. Auscultate the child's lungs when he or she is not crying.
    d. Obtain a tympanic or temporal temperature.

38. Which of the following assessments about a patient's cough should be documented?
    a. Whether it is productive or nonproductive
    b. Color of sputum
    c. Time that each cough occurred
    d. Respiratory rate prior to the patient coughing
    e. Approximate amount of sputum
    f. Sputum specimen obtained after each cough
    g. Consistency of sputum

39. A patient's face and neck are swollen. When you palpate the area, you feel crackling beneath your fingers. What could this be an indication of?
    a. The patient has fluid beneath the skin of her face and neck.
    b. The patient has developed a tension pneumothorax.
    c. The patient has air from the lungs in the subcutaneous tissue.
    d. The patient has fluid in the chest cavity resulting in a pleural effusion.

40. A 54-year-old hospitalized patient with a diagnosis of congestive heart failure is normally quite alert and easygoing. Now he seems unsure of the time of day. When you tell him it is early evening, he becomes irritated with you. What concern would you have?
    a. The patient could be developing early Alzheimer's disease with a rapid onset.
    b. The patient may have an undetected brain injury causing personality changes.
    c. The patient may be developing hypoxia and further assessment is indicated.
    d. The patient may be having a CVA (stroke) and should be sent to the operating room as soon as possible.

41. A patient from Africa has a positive reading after a TB skin test. What is the significance of this?
 a. The patient has active tuberculosis and should be quarantined.
 b. The patient may have a false-positive result as a result of a malaria vaccine but needs follow-up testing.
 c. The patient may have a resistant form of pneumonia and should have more testing.
 d. The patient may have asthma or another type of restrictive lung disease and should have pulmonary function tests.

42. Which respiratory diagnostic test measures the amount of air that can be exhaled with force?
 a. Pulmonary function tests
 b. Peak flow
 c. Chest x-ray
 d. TB skin test

43. Why is a patient at risk for pneumonia if he or she is unable to get out of bed?
 a. Many bacteria and viruses are present in the hospital that could lead to pneumonia.
 b. Mucus pools in the lungs, providing a favorable environment for bacterial growth.
 c. When on bedrest, the patient is more prone to develop asthma, which can lead to pneumonia.
 d. The need for supplemental oxygen increases with bedrest, which then increases the risk of developing pneumonia.

44. Which is true of administering nebulizer treatments?
 a. Medications must be mixed with saline carefully to avoid overdosing.
 b. A physician's order is required before a nebulizer treatment can be given.
 c. The medication is given as an inhaled spray mixed with oxygen.
 d. The medication can only be delivered using a mask, making it difficult for patients with claustrophobia to use nebulizers.

45. What will you teach your home health client regarding oxygen safety?
 a. Put up 'No Smoking' signs on the doors to the house.
 b. Keep the oxygen source in a different room from any open flame heaters, fireplaces, or stoves.
 c. You may burn candles in the same room as the oxygen source because it is a small flame.
 d. Use cotton and linen sheets and gowns, not synthetics, to decrease static electricity.

46. Which order for a patient with severe chronic obstructive pulmonary disease would you question?
 a. Eat a high-protein, low-carbohydrate diet.
 b. Have oxygen continuously at 5 L/min per nasal cannula.
 c. Turn, cough, and deep-breathe every 2 hours.
 d. Ambulate in hall once per day with E-cylinder.

47. Why do patients with chronic lung disease have difficulty eating and bathing?
 a. They must use the same muscles for breathing as they use to eat and bathe, making it difficult to do both.
 b. Chronic lung disease causes loss of appetite and lack of interest in hygiene.
 c. Mental changes that go with hypoxia cause the patient to forget to eat or bathe.
 d. Patients with chronic illnesses have little control in their lives, so they choose to have control over eating and bathing.

48. A patient with COPD is having difficulty eating. What might you suggest to help her?
 a. Encourage the use of low-carbohydrate and high-protein and high-calorie meal supplements.
 b. Encourage the patient to eat a high-carbohydrate snack every 2 hours to increase energy reserves.
 c. Have the family prepare foods that do not have to be chewed to decrease the patient's shortness of breath during meals.
 d. Encourage the patient to eat frequent, small meals rather than three large ones.

49. You are assisting a patient who has chronic lung disease with a shower. The patient is very short of breath. Which of the following will you do to make the experience easier for the patient?
 a. Make sure that the patient spends less than 20 minutes on undressing, bathing, and redressing.
 b. Place a chair or bench in the shower so the patient can sit down while being washed.
 c. Assist the patient into a terrycloth robe to absorb water, rather than having him or her dry off with a towel.
 d. Remove the oxygen while the patient is showering to encourage him or her to bathe quickly.

50. A patient must be suctioned frequently through the nose. Which of these actions by the nurse would be most helpful?
 a. Placing a nasopharyngeal airway and suctioning through it
 b. Ensuring that a humidifier is in the room to thin secretions
 c. Providing oxygen by mask rather than by nasal cannula
 d. Using petroleum jelly to lubricate the suction catheter

51. What is the advantage of using a Yankauer suction device, or tonsil tip, to suction the patient's mouth?
    a. It can be easily used in both the nose and mouth.
    b. If the patient bites down, the device will not be damaged and can still be used for suction.
    c. It does not have to be rinsed with sterile saline before and after suctioning.
    d. It does not require that the nurse wear gloves because it is contained in a sterile sleeve.

52. A patient with a tracheostomy who is not connected to a ventilator begins to choke when drinking water. What action will you take?
    a. Inflate the cuff if it is not fully inflated.
    b. Perform the Heimlich maneuver.
    c. Call the physician stat.
    d. Make the patient NPO.

53. The purpose of inserting chest tubes is to:
    a. Remove necrotic tissue from the chest cavity.
    b. Move the heart and lungs away from the center of the chest.
    c. Reestablish negative pressure within the pleural space.
    d. All of these are purposes of chest tubes.

54. What is/are the purpose(s) of the water seal in a chest tube drainage unit?
    a. To reestablish the negative pressure in the pleural space
    b. To prevent air from entering the pleural space through the chest tube
    c. To provide a method for blood and drainage to leave the pleural space
    d. To provide a method for air to leave the pleural space

Match the oxygen sources and delivery devices with their descriptions.

_____55. Oxygen concentrator

_____56. Piped-in oxygen

_____57. Liquid oxygen

_____58. T-piece

_____59. Tracheostomy collar

_____60. Venturi mask

_____61. Partial rebreathing mask

_____62. Nonrebreathing mask

a. Mask with bag attached that traps carbon dioxide for rebreathing to lower pH levels
b. Oxygen that is kept cold in a large, barrel-shaped container
c. A mask that contains a plastic valve between the tubing from the oxygen source and the mask, which allows a precise mix of room air and oxygen to equal a specific percentage of oxygen delivered to the patient
d. A device that removes some oxygen from room air and concentrates it for delivery of up to 4 L/min; requires electricity to work
e. Found in health-care facilities with a wall outlet above the bed; flowmeter is inserted into the wall to access oxygen within the pipe
f. Prevents the patient from rebreathing any exhaled air; it escapes through a one-way valve that does not allow room air to enter; only delivery device that can provide 100% oxygen when set at 15 L/min
g. Delivers highly humidified oxygen through large tubing; rests over the tracheostomy with an elastic band that goes around the neck
h. Attaches to the flange of the tracheostomy; oxygen flows from one side to the trachea; exhaled air exits through the open end

Write a brief explanation of the significance of sputum color.

63. Pink and bubbly = _____

64. Yellow or green = _____

65. Clear or white = _____

66. Gray or black = _____

67. Rust colored = _____

Part 4. Application and Critical Thinking Questions

Choose the correct answer(s). More than one answer may be correct. Select all that apply.

68. You are caring for a patient who has an asthma attack. He is having difficulty breathing and is very anxious. Which would be the most helpful for you to say at this point?
    a. "You are just anxious. Try to relax and breathe more deeply and slowly."
    b. "I think you will be just fine in a minute. Your blood-work all looked good this morning."
    c. "Somebody get help quick! This patient is having an asthma attack!"
    d. "I won't leave you like this. Breathe with me...in, out, in, out. That's good."

Situation Questions

Write a brief answer to the following questions.

▶ *Situation: Questions 69 through 71 refer to this scenario.*

Your grandfather has emphysema, a chronic obstructive lung disease. You have healthy lungs.

69. What is the chemical stimulus for you to breathe?

_____

_____

_____

_____

70. What is the chemical stimulus for your grandfather to breathe?

_____

_____

_____

_____

71. Your grandfather is receiving continuous supplemental oxygen at 2 L/min/NC. Your grandmother wants you to "turn it up because he is having trouble getting his breath." How will you respond?

_____

_____

_____

_____

▶ *Situation: Question 72 refers to this scenario.*

You are using a pulse oximeter on a patient who has dark red nail polish on all of her fingernails. You remove it from one nail, but the reading is still low at 86%. The patient is in no distress and is not short of breath.

72. What is your next step?

_____

_____

_____

▶ *Situation: Question 73 refers to this scenario.*

Your patient has just returned from surgery and is not yet fully conscious. The patient is not on a ventilator but is breathing on his own.

73. What can you do to prevent airway obstruction?

_____

_____

_____

_____

◗ *Scenario: Questions 74 through 75 refer to this scenario.*

You are caring for Nicole Whitely, a 24-year-old patient with severe asthma. She has had a tracheostomy in place for 2 weeks because of a severe asthma attack. She coughed out her tracheostomy because it had not been secured well by the nurse on the previous shift. You have called for help. Another nurse is providing breaths for her with an Ambu bag, and the physician is on the way. You are preparing for emergency reinsertion of the tracheostomy.

74. What equipment and supplies will you need?

_____

_____

_____

_____

75. What assessments will you make on Nicole after she is stable with the tracheostomy tube reinserted?

_____

_____

_____

_____

Documentation Exercise

You are caring for Nick Woods. He is a 28-year-old with a traumatic chest injury from a motor vehicle accident. He has both a pneumothorax and a hemothorax as a result. He is in Room 614. His ID is #432678. His date of birth is 6/10/88. He was admitted on 5/9/17. Today is 5/12/17 and he was moved out of ICU and onto your nursing unit at 1120. He has two chest tubes in place and is on oxygen at 4 L/min/NC. He is alert and oriented. He has several fractured ribs and is receiving pain medication for that.

You read the previous documentation of his chest tubes. You see that the escaping air in the water seal chamber was a 7 on admission to the ICU, then a 5 on 5/11/17, and a 4 today. This tells you that his pneumothorax is resolving. You also note that his chest tube output has been between 250 and 300 mL for each 24-hour period since admission to the ICU.

When you go in to assess Nick at 1430, you find that he is somewhat short of breath. He tells you that he just returned to bed from using the urinal. His respirations are 24/min and somewhat labored. He voided 300 mL of dark amber urine. As he turns to his left side in the bed, you observe that he has had 200 mL of red output in his chest tube in the past hour. When you began your shift, the chest tube drainage was marked at 850 mL by the off-going nurse at 0700. Now, at 1430, the fluid in the collection chamber is at 1300 mL, 200 mL of which has been since 1330. You see bubbles in the water-seal chamber, but it remains at a 4. You check all of his chest tube connections and find no problems. You listen to his lungs and note that he has decreased breath sounds in the lower lobe on the right side. When you assess his vital signs, you find that his BP is lower than it was at 1200 vital signs. It has dropped from 138/86 to 118/74. You decide to call the physician immediately because you are concerned about a possible hemorrhage in this patient.

76. Document your assessment and actions on the nurse's notes (Fig. 28-1) and the intake and output sheet (Fig. 28-2).

| Patient _____ |
| ID# _____ RM _____ |
| BD _____-_____-_____ |
| Admit _____-_____-_____ |
| Physician _____ |

Mission Regional Hospital

Date	Time	Nurse's Notes

Figure 28.1 Nurse's note.

Patient _____   Date _____   Shift _____

Intake	Output

Figure 28.2 Intake and output record.

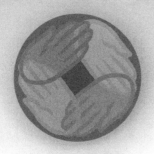

CHAPTER

Fluids, Electrolytes, and Acid-Base Balance

29

Name:	
Date:	
Course:	
Instructor:	

Part 1. Key Terms Review

Match the following Key Term(s) or italicized words from your text with the correct description.

_____ 1. Aldosterone

_____ 2. Antidiuretic hormone

_____ 3. Dehydration

_____ 4. Extracellular compartment

_____ 5. Fluid-volume deficit

_____ 6. Interstitial space

_____ 7. Intracellular compartment

_____ 8. Intravascular space

_____ 9. Third-spacing

_____10. Ascites

a. Contains body fluid that is located outside the cells; includes both fluid between the cells and inside the blood vessels

b. When osmoreceptors in the hypothalamus detect increased blood osmolality, the posterior pituitary releases this hormone, which tells kidney tubules to increase water reabsorption

c. Results with equal loss of fluid and electrolytes; water-to-solute ratio must remain balanced even though there is a loss; also called *hypovolemia*

d. The area that holds the fluid that is inside each tissue cell

e. Fluids are shifted to areas where they do not contribute to fluid and electrolyte balance between ICF and ECF

f. Area holding the fluids between and around cells

g. Loss of fluid only; results in an increase of electrolyte concentration in the remaining body fluid

h. Distention of the abdomen resulting from fluid collection in the peritoneal cavity

i. Area that holds the plasma

j. Mineralocorticoid that regulates fluid and electrolyte balance by stimulating the kidneys to retain more sodium and excrete potassium

243

Fill in the blank with the correct Key Term(s) or italicized words from your text.

11. A substance that either binds with a strong acid to decrease acidity or binds with a strong base to decrease alkalinity of the body is known as a _____.

12. A condition where the pH of body fluids is below 7.35, caused by either inadequate alkalinity or excessive acidity (or both), is called _____.

13. The movement of either solute or solvent (most commonly solute particles) that flows over naturally from an area of higher concentration into an area of lower concentration is termed _____.

14. The main anion in extracellular fluid, controlled by the kidneys, whose primary function is to serve as an alkaline buffer in regulating the acid-base balance of the blood is _____.

15. The process in which water moves through a semipermeable membrane from the fluid that is lowest in solute concentration to the side where the fluid is highest in solute concentration in an effort to balance the concentration of solutes on both sides of the membrane is known as _____.

16. When there are either excessive alkaline substances, also known as bases, or inadequate acidic substances, it causes the condition known as _____.

17. The term designating the passage of fluid through a partial barrier separating the fluid from certain particles that are too large to pass through the semipermeable membrane is _____.

18. The unit of measurement most commonly used for reporting of serum electrolyte results is mEq, which stands for _____.

19. _____ is the liquid portion of the blood that remains after removing the blood cells, is approximately 90% water, and normally contains proteins that are too large to pass through the semipermeable capillary walls.

Part 2. Connection Questions

Choose the correct answer(s). In some questions, more than one answer is correct. Select all that apply.

20. The average full-term infant's body consists of which of the following percentages of water weight?
    a. 60% to 65%
    b. 50% to 55%
    c. 65% to 80%
    d. 65% to 70%
    e. 55% to 60%

21. The average older adult body is approximately _____ water weight?
    a. 60% to 65%
    b. 50% to 55%
    c. 65% to 80%
    d. 65% to 70%
    e. 55% to 60%

22. How does an average adult female's percentage of water weight compare to the average adult male's?
    a. They are the same percentage.
    b. The female's is 5% to 10% less than the male's.
    c. The male's is 5% to 10% less than the female's.
    d. The male's is 30% higher than the female's.
    e. The female is 50% compared with the male at 70%.

23. Which of the following age groups is the exception that falls outside the range of percentages in which all the other age groups will fit?
    a. Full-term infants
    b. Adult males
    c. Premature infants
    d. Adult females
    e. Children
    f. Older adults

24. Which of the following spaces contains approximately two thirds of the body's fluids?
    a. Intracellular
    b. Interstitial
    c. Intravascular
    d. Extracellular

25. The effects of third-spacing include which of the following?
    a. Increasing the plasma volume, which results in diuresis, thereby ridding the body of the excess fluid
    b. Increasing the volume of fluid in the interstitial spaces, possibly causing excessive edema
    c. Lowering the solute concentration of the interstitial fluid, causing excessive amounts of water to move into the cells, resulting in overhydration and possible rupture of the cells, better known as *cellular death*
    d. Lowering the volume of the blood, thereby lowering the blood pressure

26. Water is necessary to support life because of its many functions. Which of the following is(are) not a function of water?
    a. Water helps to maintain the body's level of heat and cold.
    b. Water transports electrolytes, minerals, and vitamins to all the individual cells throughout the body.
    c. Water begins the cascade of enzyme-induced conversions, the end product of which stimulates the adrenal cortex to produce its primary mineralocorticoid.
    d. Water transports waste products from the cells to the blood.
    e. Water acts as a cushion for organs such as the brain and spinal cord.
    f. Water molecules bind with oxygen molecules to form carbonic acid.

27. Which of the following electrolytes is key to fluid moving in and out of cells and capillaries?
    a. Calcium
    b. Chloride
    c. Potassium
    d. Sodium

28. Which of the following accurately describes the effects that ADH has in the body?
    a. It signals the kidneys to increase diuresis, pulling more water from the body to be excreted as urine.
    b. It suppresses urine production, thereby increasing the concentration of the urine.
    c. It directs the kidneys to increase water reabsorption.
    d. It regulates the body's water level independently of solutes.

29. ANF is another hormone that affects the body's water level. Which of the following statements regarding ANF is(are) not accurate?
    a. ANF is produced by the atrium of the heart.
    b. ANF's production is signaled when baroreceptors detect abnormally low pressure, meaning that blood volume is too low.
    c. ANF inhibits renin production by the kidneys.
    d. ANF causes sodium to be retained by the kidneys.
    e. The end result of ANF increases water loss through the kidneys.

30. The average adult needs to drink how much water each day?
    a. 0.5 L
    b. 1 L
    c. 1.5 to 2 L
    d. 2 to 3 L
    e. 3 to 4 L

31. Which of the following would be likely to need more water than the average adult?
    a. Newborn infant
    b. Premature newborn
    c. Seven-year-old boy
    d. Elderly woman
    e. Pregnant woman

32. The body can make how much water from hydrogen and oxygen each day?
    a. 50 mL
    b. 100 to 300 mL
    c. 300 to 400 mL
    d. 10 to 100 mL
    e. 500 mL

33. An older adult, or senior, with cardiac disease such as congestive heart failure is at risk for fluid-volume overload. Which of the following interventions might be appropriate?
    a. Provide some coffee or tea as part of daily fluid intake.
    b. Restrict fluids.
    c. Increase salt intake.
    d. Monitor daily weights.

34. If you suspect that a patient has fluid-volume depletion, which of the following test results would confirm your suspicion?
    a. High urine-specific gravity
    b. Low urine-specific gravity
    c. Decreased hemoglobin and hematocrit
    d. Increased hemoglobin and hematocrit

35. Hypervolemia is volume excess. Which of the following statements is(are) true regarding hypervolemia?
    a. Most fluid-volume excess is caused by drinking too much water and other fluids.
    b. Hypervolemia may be caused by infusion of too much sodium chloride intravenously.
    c. Generally, most hypervolemia is a result of retention of sodium and water in the interstitial spaces and intravascular compartment.
    d. Certain illnesses, such as kidney disease, may cause the body to excrete sodium, which increases the vascular volume.
    e. All causes of hypervolemia result in decreased urinary output and expansion of fluid volume within the intravascular and interstitial spaces.

36. Which of the following signs and symptoms may point toward a fluid-volume excess?
    a. Pulse rate of 56
    b. Elevated blood pressure
    c. Clear lung fields
    d. Weight gain of 4 pounds in 2 days
    e. Edema of extremities
    f. Rales
    g. Respiratory rate of 26 per minute
    h. Decrease in pulse volume

37. Which of the following interventions might be applicable for a patient with fluid-volume excess?
    a. Administration of a diuretic ordered by the physician
    b. Encouraging consumption of a high-sodium diet ordered by the physician
    c. Auscultating the breath sounds every 4 hours to detect adventitious breath sounds
    d. Monitoring daily weights
    e. Assessing the SpO_2 every 4 hours, noting decreases
    f. Encouraging oral fluid intake of at least 1800 mL/day
    g. Monitoring I/O, estimating the volume of fluid intake and the volume of urine produced

38. It is pertinent that you monitor which of the following laboratory results on a patient to whom you are giving furosemide, a loop diuretic?
    a. Hemoglobin
    b. White blood cell count
    c. Urinalysis
    d. Potassium level

39. How are electrolytes measured in the blood and in foods?
    a. They are measured in mEq in both blood and food.
    b. They are measured in mg in both blood and food.
    c. They are measured in mEq in blood and mg in food.
    d. They are measured in mg in blood and mEq in food.

40. Your patient is taking furosemide routinely and tends to run a low serum K+ level even though the physician has prescribed K+ supplementation and the patient reports taking it faithfully. Which of the following foods would you recommend the patient add to his diet to assist in maintaining normal K+ levels?
    a. Baked potatoes
    b. Whole-grain bread
    c. Bananas
    d. Oranges
    e. Apricots
    f. Halibut
    g. Green beans
    h. White beans

41. Your knowledge of which of the following pieces of data regarding potassium takes highest priority?
    a. Never give KCl IV push.
    b. Never administer potassium chloride by direct intravenous route.
    c. KCl given IV push can cause fatal cardiac arrhythmias.
    d. Yes, this is a trick question. All of the above choices are essentially the same, but you probably will be able to remember to never give KCl direct IV push.

42. Ionized calcium is pertinent for which of the following bodily functions?
    a. Delivery of glucose into the cells
    b. Transmission of electrical impulses along nerve pathways
    c. Coagulation of blood
    d. Normal bowel function
    e. Muscle contraction and relaxation

43. The blood's bicarbonate level is controlled by which system(s)?
    a. Respiratory system
    b. Renal system
    c. Buffer system
    d. Respiratory, renal, and buffer systems

44. A patient with hypermagnesium may exhibit which of the following signs or symptoms?
    a. Hypoactive nervous system responses
    b. Hyperactive nervous system responses
    c. Increased respiratory rate
    d. Decreased respiratory rate
    e. Generally depressed neuromuscular junctions
    f. Generally stimulated neuromuscular junctions

45. Some of the following statements are accurate with regard to administration of some forms of IV calcium for hypocalcemia. Which statement(s) is(are) not accurate?
    a. IV infusion of calcium can cause bradycardia.
    b. It is pertinent to ambulate the patient who is receiving IV infusions of calcium to help metabolize the calcium.
    c. The IV site should be assessed every 2 hours for extravasation.
    d. If infused too rapidly, intravenous infusion of calcium can result in death of the patient.

46. A patient who consumes a diet that is deficient in vitamin D may be at risk for deficiency of which of the following?
    a. Calcium
    b. Potassium
    c. Phosphorus
    d. Magnesium

47. Which electrolyte(s) has(have) an inverse relationship with bicarbonate?
    a. Sodium
    b. Chloride
    c. Potassium
    d. Magnesium

48. Which of the following electrolytes is(are) controlled by aldosterone?
    a. Sodium
    b. Chloride
    c. Potassium
    d. Magnesium

49. Which electrolyte(s) is(are) necessary for the formation of hydrochloric acid found in the stomach?
    a. Sodium
    b. Chloride
    c. Potassium
    d. Magnesium

Part 3. Review Questions

Fill in the blank with the correct term(s) from your text.

50. The typical Western diet does not include adequate levels of the electrolytes _____ and _____ to maintain optimal health.

51. Approximately half of the total serum calcium is _____, meaning that it is physiologically active for use in various body functions.

52. Hypocalcemia can be responsible for bleeding problems and _____ (select either *high* or *low*) blood pressure.

53. When there is a low magnesium level or a high calcium level, you will want to assess for a low _____ level.

54. The Institute of Medicine recommends that an average adult needs _____ milligrams of potassium per day for optimal health.

55. _____ may be administered to reduce the serum level of potassium when it reaches dangerously high levels.

56. The electrolyte _____ works at the neuromuscular junctions, producing somewhat of a sedative effect, reducing the excitability and twitching of the muscles.

57. Magnesium, _____, and potassium levels are closely related: When blood level of one is down, the other two are likely to also be decreased.

58. The "p" and the "H" (as in *pH*) stand for _____.

59. The pH of human blood must stay within a very narrow range to support life. That narrow range of pH of human blood is between _____ and _____.

60. The pH scale measures or compares the numbers of two components that are present in a solution and by their presence determines the solution's acidity or alkalinity. Those two components are _____ and _____.

61. The chemical symbols for the two components in question 60 are _____ and _____, respectively.

62. The chemical symbol for the weak acid known as carbonic acid is _____.

Data: The pH scale goes from 0 to 14. Questions 63 through 67 refer to this scale. For questions 63 through 65, fill in each blank with the correct numbers from the scale.

63. On this scale, neutral is considered to be at _____.

64. An alkaline pH would be one that falls between

    _____ and _____.

65. An acidic pH would be one that falls between

    _____ and _____.

For questions 66 and 67, fill in each blank with the correct term.

66. An acidic pH would have more _____

    ions than _____ ions.

67. An alkaline pH would have more _____

    ions than _____ ions.

For questions 68 and 69, fill in each blank with the correct chemical symbol.

68. What is the chemical symbol for bicarbonate?

    _____

69. What is the chemical symbol for sodium bicarbonate?

    _____

Indicate whether the following statements are True (T) or False (F).

_____70. Dilutional hyponatremia can be inadvertently caused by medical health-care providers by administration of multiple tap-water enemas, repeated irrigation of nasogastric tubes with tap or distilled water, and infusion of excessive sodium-free IV fluids.

_____71. A patient's hemoglobin and hematocrit will show an immediate drop below normal as soon as the patient begins to hemorrhage.

_____72. Blood urea nitrogen (BUN) may appear to be elevated as a result of a fluid-volume excess.

_____73. In renal failure, the kidneys do a poor job of filtering the excess potassium from the blood, which raises the serum level to problematic levels.

_____74. Other metabolic processes other than diseases of the kidneys can alter acid-base balance.

Part 4. Application and Critical Thinking Questions

Write a brief answer to the following questions.

▶ *Scenario: Questions 75 through 78 refer to this scenario.*

Lynda Smith, a respiratory therapist at the hospital where you work, has been ill with a viral gastrointestinal flu, with nausea and vomiting for several days. On assessment you expect to find signs of dehydration rather than fluid-volume deficit.

75. List at least three assessment findings that you might see that would support your theory of dehydration.

    _____

    _____

    _____

    _____

    _____

76. Explain how fluid-volume depletion and dehydration are different.

_____

_____

_____

_____

_____

77. Explain why seniors are more at risk for dehydration than the average adult.

_____

_____

_____

_____

78. How can serum electrolyte levels be within normal range if the patient has fluid-volume deficit? Give an example when this might happen.

_____

_____

_____

_____

_____

▶ *Scenario: Question 79 refers to this scenario.*

You are caring for Ramon Cortez, who has just been admitted for fluid-volume deficit and needs intravenous fluid replacement. On taking Mr. Cortez's medical history, you find that he has had congestive heart failure for 4 to 5 years. You know that this increases his risk for fluid-volume overload, even though he does need fluid replacement therapy.

79. What nursing interventions should you perform to ensure that he does not develop fluid-volume overload?

_____

_____

_____

_____

_____

_____

▶ *Scenario: Questions 80 and 81 refer to this scenario.*

80. You are caring for Shandy Baggs, who has just been admitted with fluid-volume deficit. She reports that she has been working outside in temperatures around 105°F for the past 2 days. What assessment findings do you anticipate you will find?

_____

_____

_____

_____

_____

_____

_____

81. What interventions would be appropriate for Shandy?

_____

_____

_____

_____

_____

_____

_____

_____

▶ *Scenario: Question 82 refers to this scenario.*

The patient in Room 214 is suffering from renal failure and fluid-volume overload.

82. What laboratory results might you expect to find that would be indicative of fluid overload? Discuss at least four.

_____

_____

_____

_____

_____

_____

83. If a potassium (K+) supplement contains 20 mEq, it would be considered equal to how much K+ in food sources?

_____

_____

84. When mixing an electrolyte in less than a 1,000-mL bag of IV fluid, what nursing action should be performed to help prevent inadvertent administration errors?

_____

_____

_____

_____

85. When you add KCl to a 1,000-mL bag of IV solution, it is pertinent that you do what? Explain your answer.

_____

_____

_____

_____

86. Explain how calcium is regulated between the blood and the skeletal system.

_____

_____

_____

_____

87. Describe what is meant by *pathological fracture*.

_____

_____

For questions 88 through 99, use the process listed in Chapter 29, Box 29-8, of your textbook to evaluate the pH, CO_2, and HCO_3 levels. Determine whether the arterial blood gases are WNL (within normal limits), respiratory alkalosis or acidosis, metabolic alkalosis or acidosis, or a combination of the two. (Normal ranges: pH = 7.35–7.45; CO_2 = 35–45; HCO_3 = 22–26.)

88. pH = 7.45 CO_2 = 41 HCO_3 = 24 _____

89. pH = 7.31 CO_2 = 48 HCO_3 = 27 _____

90. pH = 7.48 CO_2 = 44 HCO_3 = 31 _____

91. pH = 7.44 CO_2 = 47 HCO_3 = 27 _____

92. pH = 7.50 CO_2 = 33 HCO_3 = 29 _____

93. pH = 7.30 CO_2 = 40 HCO_3 = 18 _____

94. pH = 7.29 CO_2 = 51 HCO_3 = 21 _____

95. pH = 7.47 CO_2 = 38 HCO_3 = 30 _____

96. pH = 7.28 CO_2 = 55 HCO_3 = 25 _____

97. pH = 7.53 CO_2 = 32 HCO_3 = 24 _____

98. pH = 7.36 CO_2 = 49 HCO_3 = 28 _____

99. pH = 7.25 CO_2 = 36 HCO_3 = 17 _____

Documentation Exercise

▶ *Scenario:*

The patient's name is Sally Field (but she is not the movie star). Her hospital ID is #34623 and she is in Room 209. Her BD is 7/19/52, and she was admitted on 9/1/17. Today's date is 9/2/17 and the time is 1900. Ms. Field has congestive heart failure and has been placed on restricted fluid intake of 1000 mL/24 hours, or 500 mL per 12-hour shift. Her current vital signs are 158/86, T 99.2 taken orally, P 102 regular and strong, and respirations are 28 per minute and are regular and even. Auscultation of her breath sounds still finds rales in LLL, LUL, RUL, RML, and RLL. Her skin is pink, warm, and dry. Her oral mucosa is pink. Her skin turgor is elastic. She denies any pain or discomfort but does report that she becomes very short of breath any time she moves about. At this time she is lying supine. Her total intake for this shift was 500 mL, and she had 660 mL of clear pale-yellow urine. She did not have a BM. She has oxygen on at 4 L/min being delivered by a nasal cannula. Her oxygen saturation level is 93%.

100. Use a nurse's note form (Fig. 29-1) and document these data in an orderly and succinct manner. This is your last entry for your 7 a.m. to 7 p.m. shift. Be certain to sign your name and credentials.

Patient _____		
ID# _____ RM _____		**Mission Regional Hospital**
BD _____-_____-_____		
Admit _____-_____-_____		
Physician _____		

Date	Time	Nurse's Notes

Figure 29.1 Nurse's note.

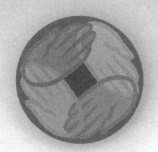

Bowel Elimination and Care

Name: _____
Date: _____
Course: _____
Instructor: _____

Part 1. Key Terms Review

Match the following Key Term(s) or italicized words from your text with the correct description.

_____ 1. Constipation

_____ 2. Diarrhea

_____ 3. Guaiac

_____ 4. Distention

_____ 5. Incontinence

_____ 6. Steatorrhea

_____ 7. Tenesmus

_____ 8. Occult blood

_____ 9. Flatus

_____10. Defecation

a. Increased rectal pressure and feeling of need to defecate

b. Process of bowel elimination

c. Less frequent, hard-formed stools that are difficult to expel

d. Stool containing an abnormally high amount of undigested fat

e. Several liquid or watery stools per day

f. A gas produced when intestinal bacteria interact with chyme

g. Being stretched out or inflated

h. A test done to determine presence of hidden blood

i. Blood that is hidden or not visible to the naked eye

j. The lack of voluntary control of elimination of urine or stool

Fill in the blank with the correct Key Term(s) or italicized words from your text.

11. The mouth or opening of an ostomy is called the

_____.

12. The diversion created by bringing a portion of the large intestine, or colon, to the outside of the body through the abdominal wall is called a _____.

13. The blockage of the movement of contents through the intestines by a bulk of very hard stool is known as a

_____.

14. Commonly administered to relieve a patient of excessive intestinal gas is the _____ enema.

15. The diversion made by bringing the ileum to the outside of the body through the abdominal wall for elimination is called an _____.

16. A special type of medicated solution administered rectally for the purpose of lowering a very high potassium level is known as a _____.

17. Blood from higher in the digestive tract, such as the stomach, that has been partially digested and has a distinctive old blood odor and a black, tarry appearance is known as _____.

18. The rhythmic, wavelike contractions that begin in the esophagus and continue throughout the gastrointestinal (GI) tract to the rectum is called _____.

19. Another name for the siphon enema is a _____.

20. Residual bacteria that live in the intestinal tract and whose purpose is to prevent infection and maintain health are called _____.

Part 2. Connection Questions

Choose the correct answer(s). In some questions, more than one answer is correct. Select all that apply.

21. In the GI tract, a food bolus is converted into a semiliquid mass of partly digested food and digestive secretions known as:
    a. Effluent
    b. Chyme
    c. Emulsion
    d. A bezoar

22. You are administering an enema to a female patient who is constipated. You notice the patient's skin is pale and a little moist. You take the pulse and obtain a rate of 44 bpm. What do you suspect is occurring?
    a. She is having a vagal response.
    b. She has a fecal impaction.
    c. She is hemorrhaging internally.
    d. This is a normal reaction to an enema when one is so full of feces.

23. During your initial shift assessment of Bhojraj Bellerive, one of your assigned patients for the day, he reports that he has not had a bowel movement since the day before yesterday. You know that the maximum time that you should allow a patient to go without having a bowel movement is:
    a. 1 day
    b. 2 days
    c. 3 days
    d. 7 days

24. Carlos Cuellar, a patient on your wing, rings his call light and tells you that he has had a bowel movement and you can now collect the stool specimen for ova and parasites. You assess the stool as you collect the specimen and find that the stool does not appear normal. Which of the following descriptions of feces would not be normal?
    a. Moderate amounts of soft-formed, dark brown feces
    b. Several small, hard, pellet-like, brown pieces of feces
    c. Large amount of cylindrical-shaped light brown feces
    d. Small amount of formed medium brown feces

25. While caring for a 2-day-old male newborn you check the baby's diaper and find that he has had a bowel movement. While you change the diaper you assess the stool for abnormal characteristics. The stool is somewhat shiny and black. It is only semiformed and is very sticky, making it difficult to clean off the baby's skin. You know that:
    a. The stool is normal meconium and that there is no need for concern.
    b. Black, tarry stools indicate bleeding of the GI tract and you should phone the physician immediately to report the ominous sign.
    c. Breastfed babies commonly have black, tarry stools and there is no need for concern.
    d. The iron in the infant's formula should not cause black stools and you need to report the abnormal stool.

26. While assisting a patient who has had a bowel movement off of the bedpan, you observe that there is a large amount of bright red blood in the semiliquid feces. You can even smell the blood. You immediately report to the physician that the patient has had:
    a. A bowel movement containing occult blood
    b. Steatorrhea
    c. A bowel movement with melena
    d. A bowel movement with frank blood

27. Dr. Ruker has ordered that Chin Dong's stool be tested for hidden blood. You know to complete the laboratory requisition for a(n):
    a. Guaiac test
    b. Culture and sensitivity
    c. Ova and parasites
    d. Hemoccult test

28. Sandy Leitner, a postoperative patient who underwent an abdominal hysterectomy 2 days ago, complains that she is becoming constipated. This does not surprise you because:
    a. Her activity level has been less than normal because of the surgery.
    b. She has been receiving morphine for postoperative pain.
    c. Since her surgery she has only been out of bed twice the day of surgery, four times yesterday, and four times today.
    d. She had an enema the day before her surgery.

29. Factors that are known to cause diarrhea include:
    a. Allergies
    b. The natural aging process
    c. Depression
    d. Stress

30. Which of the following factors may prevent an individual from being able to consume an adequate amount of fiber in the diet?
    a. The patient eats cereal for breakfast daily.
    b. The patient has poorly fitting dentures.
    c. The patient has edentia.
    d. The patient does not like fruit.

31. Alice Gabor is a 78-year-old female patient who lives alone. She was admitted to the hospital with malnutrition and anemia. You are suspicious that she has a fecal impaction based on the fact that:
    a. She has been incontinent of small amounts of liquid stool several times today.
    b. Her bowel sounds are hyperactive in all four quadrants of her abdomen.
    c. Her last bowel movement was yesterday.
    d. She tells you that she has a bowel movement only every other day.

32. There are numerous things that you can do as a nurse that will make it easier for a patient to maintain his or her normal pattern of bowel elimination while hospitalized. Which of the following actions would be helpful?
    a. Wake the patient at 0700 each day and place the patient on the bedpan to establish a daily morning bowel movement.
    b. Encourage adequate fluid intake each day.
    c. If activity is not restricted, ambulate the patient in the hall at least three times per day.
    d. Inform the patient that you will have to administer an enema if she does not have a bowel movement as often as she does at home.

33. Which of the following information regarding fiber would be appropriate for you to teach a patient?
    a. A minimum of 25 to 30 g of fiber should be ingested daily.
    b. Many fruits and vegetables serve as good sources of dietary fiber.
    c. The fibers that can be purchased over the counter and by prescription are not effective to prevent constipation.
    d. If fiber intake has averaged less than 15 g/day, the amount of fiber should be immediately increased to 35 g/day.

Part 3. Review Questions

Choose the correct answer(s). In some questions, more than one answer is correct. Select all that apply.

34. Which direction should you direct the tip of the enema tube as you insert it into the rectum to reduce the risk for perforation?
    a. Toward the patient's umbilicus
    b. Toward the patient's spine
    c. Straight toward the patient's head
    d. Toward the patient's feet

35. Which of the following food/drink items would be appropriate after the first 24 hours that an adult has diarrhea?
    a. Bananas
    b. Piece of aged cheese
    c. Cup of hot chocolate
    d. Applesauce
    e. Small milkshake
    f. Hot cup of coffee
    g. Glass of iced tea

36. Which of the following food/drink items would be appropriate for the first 24 hours that an infant has diarrhea?
    a. Cooked carrots
    b. Bottle of Pedialyte
    c. Bottle of milk
    d. Applesauce
    e. Mashed bananas
    f. Bottle of room-temperature chamomile tea

37. Most water is absorbed in which portion of the gastrointestinal tract?
    a. Stomach
    b. Duodenum
    c. Ileum
    d. Colon

38. The proper name for the fecal material expelled from a new colostomy is:
    a. Mucoid feces
    b. Steatorrhea
    c. Effluent
    d. Diarrhea stools

39. A healthy stoma should be:
    a. A light bluish purple color
    b. Shiny and moist
    c. Cool and dry
    d. A pinkish red color

Part 4. Application and Critical Thinking Questions

Choose the correct answer(s). In some questions, more than one answer is correct. Select all that apply.

40. It is common for patients who are taking antibiotics to develop diarrhea as a result of the loss of normal flora from the intestines. Which of the following interventions would be helpful for these patients?
    a. Increase consumption of fresh fruits and vegetables.
    b. Add yogurt to the daily diet.
    c. Take lactobacillus acidophilus.
    d. Drink 4 ounces of apple juice with each meal.

41. Which of the following types of enemas would be safe to administer to infants and patients with congestive heart failure?
    a. SS enema made with tap water
    b. Saline enema
    c. Harris flush not made with saline
    d. A hypotonic solution enema

42. Before it is safe for you to delegate to the UAP the administration of an enema to a patient, it is necessary to:
    a. Ask the patient for permission.
    b. Administer the first enema yourself to ensure the patient's ability to tolerate it.
    c. Ask if the UAP can identify steps to take to prevent perforation of intestinal wall.
    d. Ensure that the UAP knows what a vagal response is.

43. What would be the first assessment you would make if the patient to whom you are administering an enema said she was feeling light-headed and faint?
    a. Assess pulse rate
    b. Assess blood pressure
    c. Ask whether or not the patient has ever felt this way before
    d. Determine whether the patient ever had an enema before
    e. Assess respiratory rate

44. You are administering an enema and have determined that the patient is having a vagal response. What should your first action be?
    a. Place patient in supine position.
    b. Apply oxygen.
    c. Call a code blue.
    d. Stop enema and remove tube from rectum.
    e. Assess vital signs.

Write a brief answer to the following questions.

45. Explain at least four of the various components that can affect an inpatient's normal bowel habits and contribute to the risk for constipation. Include at least one intervention for each component selected that would help compensate for the increased risk for constipation.

_____

_____

_____

_____

_____

_____

_____

46. What objective data should you assess and document for a new colostomy?

_____

_____

_____

_____

47. When should you empty a colostomy bag? _____

_____

Read the following brief scenario, then stop for a few moments and think about what you have just read. Picture your current self (same age and cognitive ability) as the individual described in the scenario. Concentrate on the feelings you might experience while visualizing yourself in this situation, or at least those feelings that you believe you might experience if it were the actual reality.

▶ *Scenario: Question 48 refers to this scenario.*

You are your current age and level of cognitive ability. However, there are two differences: You are unable to control your bladder or your bowels, not even part of the time, and you are not able to perform hygiene measures to clean yourself up or to even help with that process. You are lying in a hospital bed and have just been incontinent of both urine and a very large semiliquid bowel movement. The incontinence became a problem more than 24 hours ago, and you just cannot believe this is happening to you. You absolutely despise this lack of control and the dependence on others for such personal issues as toileting. Good grief! You are a student nurse. You know that cleaning up feces and urine is not something that most nurses like to do. You feel so embarrassed that you can hardly stand the thought of pressing the nurse call light. You may wish that you could become invisible so no one could see you. You may feel so anxious about calling the nurse that you think you are going to vomit all over yourself and add to the horribleness of the situation. How do you really believe you would feel? Give it a couple minutes of serious thought, visualizing the scene and feeling those feelings.

48. Describe as vividly as you can all the feelings that you imagined. Be expressive—do not mince your words. Be honest and sincere. Let the feelings flow onto your paper. Once you have completed this exercise, decide in your own mind how you can best approach each patient who requires your assistance with toileting hygiene. What can you say to the patient? How should your body language show acceptance, compassion, and understanding? What type of facial expression should you wear? In what tone of voice should you speak? Determine to remember these things as long as you live and care for others.

_____

_____

_____

_____

_____

_____

_____

_____

_____

_____

_____

_____

◗ *Scenario: Question 49 refers to this scenario.*

The patient's name is Mivin Fisher. He was born 10/5/42 and was admitted on 7/8/17. His ID is #23232. His room number is 333. Today's date is 7/8/17 and it is now 0730. You have just administered a soap suds enema 750 mL rectally. He was able to hold the enema and ambulate to the bathroom for expulsion. He has a lot of soft brown stool returned that was formed. He says that he feels so much better than he did before the enema.

49. Use a nurse's note form (Fig. 30-1) and document these data using narrative format. Be succinct and accurate.

| Patient _____ |
| ID# _____ RM _____ |
| BD _____ - _____ - _____ |
| Admit _____ - _____ - _____ |
| Physician _____ |

Mission Regional Hospital

Date	Time	Nurse's Notes

Figure 30.1 Nurse's note.

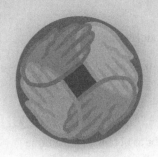

Urinary Elimination and Care

Name: _____	
Date: _____	
Course: _____	
Instructor: _____	

Part 1. Key Terms Review

Match the following Key Term(s) or italicized words from your text with the correct description.

_____ 1. Void

_____ 2. Hematuria

_____ 3. Oliguria

_____ 4. Polyuria

_____ 5. Anuria

_____ 6. Dysuria

_____ 7. Renal calculi

_____ 8. Residual urine

_____ 9. Nocturia

_____ 10. Incontinence

a. Urinary output greater than 3000 mL/day
b. Painful or difficult urination
c. Kidney stones that can occur anywhere in the renal system from the kidney to the urethra
d. Blood in the urine, either visible or microscopic
e. Waking up at night to urinate
f. Inability to control the passing of urine
g. Urinate or micturate
h. Urinary output of less than 30 mL/hr
i. Urine that remains in the bladder after the person voids
j. Absence of urine or minimal urine production

Fill in the blank with the correct Key Term(s) or italicized words from your text.

11. _____ is the process of using a machine to filter waste products and salts, and to remove excess fluid from the blood.

12. The result of comparing the weight of a substance with an equal amount of water is known as

_____.

13. The inability to empty the bladder at all or the inability to completely empty the bladder is called

    _____.

14. When urine leaks out of the bladder as a result of increased abdominal pressure, it is referred to as

    _____.

15. _____,
    also known as overactive bladder, is the inability to keep urine in the bladder long enough to get to the restroom.

16. A blood test called _____
    measures a waste product normally eliminated from the body by the kidneys. Elevated levels may reflect infection or some degree of kidney impairment.

17. A tube that remains in the bladder is an

    _____, also known
    as a double lumen catheter or a Foley catheter.

18. A single tube with holes at the end that is used to empty the bladder of residual urine or to obtain a sterile urine specimen from the bladder is a _____.

19. A _____ is used for urine to be eliminated by an alternate route rather than traveling through the bladder.

20. A _____ is caused by the presence of pathogens within the urinary tract.

Part 2. Connection Questions

Choose the correct answer(s). In some questions, more than one answer is correct. Select all that apply.

21. You are assigned to care for a patient with an indwelling catheter. A 24-hour urine collection is ordered. How will you keep the urine from deteriorating and affecting the outcome of the test?
    a. Take a labeled specimen from the drainage bag to the laboratory every 3 hours.
    b. Empty the bag every 8 hours and pour the urine into a 24-hour collection container. Keep this container refrigerated.
    c. Keep the drainage bag in a basin containing ice. Empty the drainage bag every 8 hours into the 24-hour collection container, which you are keeping in a refrigerator.
    d. Ask the patient to empty the drainage bag into an iced container whenever it contains more than 100 mL of urine.

22. Number in order the path of urine through the urinary system.
    a. ____ Bladder
    b. ____ Urinary meatus
    c. ____ Kidney
    d. ____ Urethra
    e. ____ Ureter

23. Contraction of which muscle causes the bladder to empty?
    a. Internal urinary sphincter
    b. Detrusor
    c. External urinary sphincter
    d. Peristalsis

24. Urinary sepsis is a potential complication of any UTI because:
    a. A continuous membrane lines all the structures of the urinary system.
    b. Bacteria from outside the urinary meatus can spread through the urethra to the bladder, then the ureters, and into the kidneys.
    c. Once a UTI occurs, the immune system is compromised and can no longer fight bacteria entering the blood.
    d. The total volume of a person's blood flows through the kidneys each day to be filtered, and this could allow bacteria to spread to the blood.

25. You are delegating the task of monitoring the output of an elderly male patient at risk for oliguria. He has an indwelling catheter in place. Which is the most appropriate direction for you to give to an unlicensed assistant?
    a. "Tell me if his urine output decreases."
    b. "Keep an eye on his output for me."
    c. "Check his output halfway through the shift and let me know the total."
    d. "Check his output after 2 hours. If it is not above 60 mL, let me know immediately."

26. If a patient had an order to discontinue a catheter the day after surgery, under what circumstances might you consider delaying doing so until you talk with the physician?
    a. If the patient complained of burning or discomfort because of the catheter
    b. If the patient's output is greater than 50 mL/hr
    c. If the patient's output is less than 30 mL/hr
    d. If the patient's urine is dark amber

27. Which two blood tests are most important in assessing kidney function?
    a. BUN and creatinine
    b. CBC and hematocrit
    c. BUN and hematocrit
    d. CBC and creatinine

28. Your patient has a glomerular filtration rate (GFR) of 45 mL/min over a 3-month period. What does this tell you about her kidney function?
    a. She has chronic kidney disease.
    b. She is in renal failure.
    c. She has a kidney infection.
    d. Nothing; only BUN and creatinine levels can give information about kidney function.

29. You are teaching a home care patient about self-catheterization. You know more teaching is needed when the patient states:
    a. "I will not need sterile gloves and a new sterile catheter every time I catheterize myself at home."
    b. "I will use clean gloves and wash the catheters between uses."
    c. "I do not need gloves or any special precautions because I am in my own home."
    d. "This is a clean, rather than a sterile, procedure at home."

30. Under what circumstances is it appropriate to use an indwelling catheter in a long-term care setting?
    a. If the patient has a stage I or stage II pressure ulcer
    b. If the patient has a stage III or stage IV pressure ulcer
    c. If the patient is continuously incontinent of urine and is at risk for pressure ulcers
    d. If the patient has a terminal illness
    e. If the patient has a severe impairment such that positioning and clothing changes are painful

31. Which is true of UTIs in children?
    a. They are very common, second only to respiratory infections.
    b. The symptoms are the same as those seen in adults.
    c. They occur more often in boys than in girls.
    d. They may cause a toilet-trained child to have accidents.
    e. They may cause poor feeding, vomiting, and diarrhea.

Part 3. Review Questions

Choose the correct answer(s). In some questions, more than one answer is correct. Select all that apply.

32. The kidneys filter waste products from cellular metabolism out of the blood and excrete it in the urine. Which of the following are the three most important waste products to be filtered?
    a. Urea, sodium, and potassium
    b. Creatinine, sodium, and uric acid
    c. Urea, creatinine, and uric acid
    d. Uric acid, sodium, and potassium

33. How long can a urine specimen sit unrefrigerated before it is analyzed?
    a. 30 minutes
    b. 1 hour
    c. 2 hours
    d. 3 hours

34. What is the minimum acceptable hourly urine output?
    a. 15 mL
    b. 30 mL
    c. 60 mL
    d. 90 mL

35. Some diuretics cause excessive amounts of electrolytes to be excreted. Which electrolyte is most often associated with diuretics?
    a. Sodium
    b. Potassium
    c. Chloride
    d. Bicarbonate

36. A frail elderly patient with a hip fracture has to void before surgery. Which of the following is the best way to handle this?
    a. Have the patient use a fracture pan.
    b. Have the patient use a regular bedpan.
    c. Help the patient use the bedside commode.
    d. Catheterize the patient.

37. Which of the following represents an accurate list of the factors you should assess related to urination for most patients?
    a. Color and odor of urine, amount voided at a time and in a 24-hour period, frequency and ease of urination
    b. Urine characteristics, amount voided at a time and in a 24-hour period, frequency of urination
    c. Urine characteristics, amount voided at a time and in a 24-hour period, frequency and ease of urination
    d. Urine characteristics, hourly urine output, amount voided at a time and in a 24-hour period, frequency and ease of urination, signs of fluid retention

38. Which emotional response do you think most people will experience when they need to ask for assistance with urinating?
    a. Fear related to a possible "accident"
    b. Anger related to diminished sense of self-control
    c. Shame/embarrassment related to loss of autonomy
    d. Loss of self-esteem related to inability to care for self independently

39. One quick and common way to get a lot of data about urine is by:
    a. Dipping litmus paper into the urine to determine pH
    b. Adding special stains to see if there are white blood cells in the urine
    c. Testing the urine with a multiple-pad reagent stick
    d. Observing the urine for color and clarity

40. One important nursing intervention for patients with suspected renal calculi is to:
    a. Obtain timed urine specimens.
    b. Strain the urine.
    c. Assess for hematuria.
    d. Palpate both flanks for tenderness.

41. In addition to collecting all urine passed in a 24-hour period, one of the most important steps in obtaining a 24-hour urine sample is to:
    a. Have the patient void, discard this urine, note the time, and then begin collecting.
    b. Begin the collection at 8 a.m.
    c. Make sure there is a preservative in the collection bottle.
    d. Keep the sample at room temperature.

42. Which of the following best describes the importance of monitoring intake and output?
    a. It helps determine the patient's fluid replacement needs.
    b. It can be used to correlate with daily weights.
    c. It is a good way to assess overall fluid balance.
    d. It helps determine the greatest source of fluid losses (for example, through diarrhea, insensible losses, or urine output).

43. Your patient returned from surgery (laparoscopy) 4 hours ago and complains of being unable to empty her bladder. What step should you take next?
    a. Palpate her bladder.
    b. Catheterize her.
    c. Have her drink a full glass of water and then have her try to void again.
    d. Check her vital signs.

44. Sometimes patients are not aware that they retain urine. If the residual urine volume is less than 300 mL and does not feel uncomfortable to the patient, is there any reason to try to correct the problem?
    a. Yes, because the enlarged bladder can cause pressure on other organs.
    b. Yes, because residual urine can lead to urinary tract infections.
    c. Yes, because it can cause enlarged prostate in men or urethral strictures in women.
    d. No, if the patient is not uncomfortable, a residual urine of 300 mL or less does not require treatment.

Match the type of incontinence to its causes and pathophysiology.

_____45. Stress incontinence

_____46. Urge incontinence

_____47. Overflow incontinence

_____48. Functional incontinence

_____49. Total incontinence

_____50. Neuropathic incontinence

a. Incontinence related to inability to get to the bathroom

b. The brain does not receive a message that the bladder is full

c. Incontinence related to bladder spasms and contractions

d. The bladder does not empty because of an obstruction

e. Incontinence related to weak pelvic floor muscles

f. Loss of urine with no warning

Choose the correct answer(s). In some questions, more than one answer is correct. Select all that apply.

51. Your patient has stress incontinence. Which of the following statements represent recommended treatment for this problem?
   a. Suggest the patient wear incontinence pads in a comfortable style with adequate absorbency.
   b. Tell the patient that there are medications available to help with stress incontinence and that the doctor will discuss them with her.
   c. Tell the patient to avoid abdominal exercises, which can cause stress incontinence.
   d. Tell the patient about Kegel exercises.

52. You are teaching bladder retraining to the patient with incontinence. She tries the plan and reports back to you about her progress. "I tried going to the bathroom every 2 hours like you said, but I just sit there. I'm trying now to just go when I feel the urge, which is about every 3 hours. I'm still having accidents about half the time, which is a big improvement." Which of the following statements should you make in response to the patient's comment?
   a. "That's great. Keep up that pattern. It sounds like it's working."
   b. "Waiting until you feel the urge defeats the purpose of a bladder retraining program. It sounds like you haven't really implemented the program. You should go back to trying to void every 2 hours to train your bladder to empty when you want it to."
   c. "It sounds like bladder retraining isn't working for you, but that paying greater attention to the urge to go is."
   d. "This is good information, but waiting for the urge to go is not going to retrain your bladder. Try toileting yourself every 2 1/2 hours. Do this for several days to a week and then let me know the results."

Indicate whether the following statements are True (T) or False (F).

_____ 53. An indwelling catheter has a balloon that keeps the catheter in place.

_____ 54. A straight-tipped catheter is best when catheterizing a patient with an enlarged prostate.

_____ 55. A three-way catheter is used for bladder irrigation.

_____ 56. A condom catheter is an external catheter.

_____ 57. The size of the balloon for an indwelling catheter is 5 mL.

_____ 58. In catheters, the greater the size number, the larger the catheter.

Choose the correct answer(s). In some questions, more than one answer is correct. Select all that apply.

59. You are caring for a patient who sustained a spinal cord injury 14 years ago. Two days ago, the physician inserted an indwelling urinary catheter, size 18 Fr, which is to remain in place for several weeks to allow pressure ulcers to heal. The patient has had catheters off and on for many years. You note that urine is leaking around the catheter insertion site and that the patient's meatus is getting red and irritated. Which of the following actions represents the nursing interventions most likely to resolve this situation?
   a. Request medication to calm bladder spasms, which are probably the cause of the leakage.
   b. Obtain an order to remove the current catheter and replace it with a size 22 Fr catheter.
   c. Obtain an order to replace the current catheter with a size 14 Fr catheter.
   d. Obtain an order to remove the current catheter and replace it with a condom catheter.

60. You are about to catheterize a female patient who is experiencing a decline in her physical condition. In fact, she is being transferred from your unit to the ICU. As you get ready to insert the catheter, the tip lightly brushes against the patient's leg. Which of the following possible actions should you perform next?
    a. You should get a new catheter to insert.
    b. You should report the possible contamination to the nurse in the ICU so that she can get an order for antibiotics.
    c. It is not necessary to mention it as long as you cleaned the urinary meatus according to policy.
    d. You should clean the catheter tip with alcohol or Betadine.

61. Which of the following makes catheterization difficult but represents normal anatomy in older women?
    a. The introitus is enlarged.
    b. The urinary meatus is located in the vaginal opening because of atrophy of perineal tissues.
    c. The perineal area becomes very dry.
    d. The clitoris atrophies.

62. Circumcision is:
    a. Retraction of the foreskin in males
    b. Removal of the foreskin in males
    c. Tightening of the foreskin in males
    d. Narrowing of the opening of the foreskin in males

63. You will need to push back the foreskin before catheterizing uncircumcised males. After you catheterize the patient, you should:
    a. Pull the foreskin back over the glans.
    b. Leave the foreskin retracted.
    c. Lubricate the foreskin with petroleum jelly and then replace it.
    d. Elevate the penis on a folded towel to prevent swelling of the foreskin or glans.

64. The urethra is a tube that, in males, is surrounded by prostate tissue. When the prostate enlarges, it encroaches on the urethra and narrows it. When catheterizing a male patient with an enlarged prostate, you may encounter resistance. How should you respond to this situation?
    a. Remove the catheter immediately and call the physician.
    b. Continue to try to advance the catheter. If bleeding occurs, leave the catheter in place and call the physician.
    c. Gently twist the catheter and change the position/angle of the penis to find an area of the opening large enough for the catheter to pass through.
    d. Remove the catheter and try a larger size.

65. Which of the following represents an appropriate way to maintain a urinary drainage bag?
    a. Keep the drainage bag above the level of the bladder.
    b. Tape the bag to the patient's leg.
    c. Empty the bag when it is full.
    d. Keep tubing free of kinks and coils.

66. You note that in the past 3 hours no urine has drained into your female patient's urinary collection bag. Which of the following is most likely responsible for this?
    a. Kinks in the tubing
    b. Acute renal failure
    c. Poor positioning of the drainage bag
    d. A kidney stone blocking the catheter

67. You are teaching an aide to perform catheter care. Which of the following represents an accurate statement?
    a. "Clean the perineum and a few inches of tubing using a soapy washcloth in downward strokes away from the body."
    b. "Wash the perineum with a soapy washcloth using circular motions."
    c. "Wash from the tubing 3 to 4 inches from the insertion site up toward the meatus."
    d. "Separate the labia if the patient is female and wash first on one side, then the other, and then down the middle."

68. After discontinuing an indwelling urinary catheter, what should you assess for?
    a. Swelling and discharge from the urinary meatus
    b. Whether the patient has voided within 8 hours
    c. Temporary decrease in urine output
    d. Temporary urge incontinence

Indicate whether the following statements are True (T) or False (F).

_____ 69. An infection in the bladder can spread up to infect the kidneys.

_____ 70. Urinary tract infections are more common in males than in females.

_____ 71. The alkalinity of urine helps kill bacteria.

_____ 72. Spermicides can increase the risk for urinary tract infections in women.

_____ 73. Bath salts can irritate the urethra, making it more susceptible to infection.

_____ 74. Symptoms of UTI include dysuria, urinary frequency, urgency, nocturia, low abdominal pain, and incontinence.

_____ 75. Fever, chills, malaise, nausea, vomiting, and flank pain mean the infection has most likely spread to the kidneys, causing pyelonephritis.

_____ 76. Treatment for a UTI includes rest, increased fluid intake, antibiotics, and urinary analgesics.

Part 4. Application and Critical Thinking Questions

Choose the correct answer(s). More than one answer may be correct. Select all that apply.

77. You are caring for a patient with an indwelling catheter. You have an order to discontinue the catheter this morning. The patient also has had an IV infusing at 100 mL/hr through the night. The patient is taking liquids and eating ice chips. At 0700, you notice that the output on the previous shift was 290 mL of dark amber urine and the patient's intake totaled 960 mL. Which action will you take?
    a. Get an order to irrigate the catheter prior to discontinuing it.
    b. Wait to discontinue the catheter until you can speak with the physician on morning rounds.
    c. Discontinue the catheter and discontinue the order for intake and output because the patient no longer has a tube in place.
    d. Perform a bladder scan to determine if the patient has a large amount of residual urine in the bladder.

Write a brief answer to the following questions.

▶ *Situation: Questions 78 through 80 refer to this scenario.*

You are working on a nursing unit and are caring for a male patient who has had abdominal surgery. A catheter was in place during the surgery but was discontinued in the post-anesthesia care unit (PACU). The patient attempts to void numerous times in the urinal but can only expel about 25 mL or less each time.

78. Which independent nursing measure would you implement?

_____

_____

_____

79. You gather the following assessment data: bladder is distended, patient is complaining of lower abdominal discomfort and urinary output has totaled 150 mL in 6 hours after the catheter was discontinued, and the patient is voiding frequently in very small amounts. You decide to notify the physician. What order will you expect to receive?

_____

_____

_____

80. The next day the patient continues to be unable to void more than 50 mL each time. You have performed two straight catheterizations in the past 12 hours, obtaining 650 mL the first time and 725 mL the second time. The C&S on the urine specimen you sent shows no growth on the preliminary report. What do you anticipate the physician will order next?

_____

_____

_____

▶ *Situation: Question 81 refers to this scenario.*

You answer the call light of a female patient on the opposite end of the hall than your patient assignment. You assist the patient back to bed, measure the amount of urine in the specimen pan, and record it on the intake and output sheet. Then you dump the urine into the toilet and flush it. Only then do you see the sign that says, "24-Hour Urine in Progress," with the current date and time.

81. What will you do?

_____

_____

_____

Documentation Exercise

You are caring for a patient named Suhani Mathai. Her date of birth is 1/19/72. She was admitted on May 3, 2017, with a diagnosis of multiple sclerosis and appendicitis. She is in Room 1114 and her hospital ID is #1354682. Today is May 4, 2017. She has a catheter in place when she returns from PACU. She also has an IV of D5W infusing at 60 mL/hr.

When you assume her care at 0800, you note mucous strings in the catheter tubing and her output has been 350 mL of dark amber urine over the past 3 hours. As you continue to monitor her output, you notice that the patient has no additional output over the next hour. At 0900, you notify the physician and receive orders to perform closed irrigation with normal saline. It is approximately 15 minutes later when you have gathered your supplies and perform the irrigation. You notice more mucous strings and shreds with little return of the 90 mL you used to irrigate.

In 3 more hours, you note that the urinary output is only at 450 mL. At around 1230, you decide to perform a bladder scan to see if the catheter is actually draining the bladder. It shows 300 mL of residual urine in the bladder. You again notify the physician and explain your concerns that the bladder is not draining despite the indwelling catheter. The physician gives orders to remove the existing catheter and replace it with a catheter that is one size larger.

At 1315 you discontinue the existing catheter and note the holes are plugged with mucus. You insert a size 16 French catheter and get an immediate return of 350 mL of amber urine with a few mucous shreds. You encourage your patient to increase her fluid intake and give her a large glass of cranberry juice at her request.

82. Document your assessment and actions on the nurse's notes (Fig. 31-1).

		Mission Regional Hospital
Patient _____	
ID# _____ RM _____	
BD _____-_____-_____	
Admit _____-_____-_____	
Physician _____	

Date	Time	Nurse's Notes

Figure 31.1 Nurse's note.

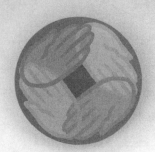

Care of Elderly Patients

| Name: _____ |
| Date: _____ |
| Course: _____ |
| Instructor: _____ |

Part 1. Key Terms Review

Match the following Key Term(s) or italicized words from your text with the correct description.

_____ 1. Cerebrovascular accident

_____ 2. Hemorrhagic stroke

_____ 3. Ischemic stroke

_____ 4. Transient ischemic attack

a. An interruption of blood flow to an area of the brain caused by a bleeding blood vessel

b. A temporary decrease in the blood supply to the brain

c. An interruption of normal blood flow to an area of the brain, resulting in death of brain tissue

d. An interruption of blood flow to an area of the brain caused by a blood clot

Fill in the blank with the correct Key Term(s) or italicized words from your text.

5. Discrimination and prejudice toward elderly people is called _____.

6. A(n) _____ occurs when a patient misinterprets sensory stimuli such as thinking an inanimate object is a human being or an animal.

7. If a confused patient tells you he or she hears a baby crying but no baby is in the area, the person is said to be having a _____.

8. A patient suffers from _____ when he or she is no longer able to care for himself or herself as a result of declining intellectual functioning.

9. When a patient gradually withdraws from social interaction, is confused, wanders, and fails to recognize family and friends, he or she is probably suffering from

_____.

10. When the lens of the eye becomes cloudy or opaque, it is referred to as a(n) _____.

11. Increased pressure in the eyeball that can lead to blindness is called _____.

12. The destruction of the area in the retina where the optic nerve attaches, leading to the loss of central vision in older adults, is called _____.

13. The technical term for heart attack is

_____.

14. A recliner with side arms, a lap belt, and wheels used for people who cannot sit unassisted is called a

_____.

15. The people who live in long-term care facilities are generally referred to as _____, not patients.

Part 2. Connection Questions

Choose the correct answer(s). In some questions, more than one answer is correct. Select all that apply.

16. An elderly patient with a hearing problem and mild confusion is not being cooperative regarding his need for a morning bath. The UAP in charge of his hygiene for the morning is frustrated and upset, and says, "Mr. Anderson isn't listening to a word I say!" Which of the following responses by the charge nurse represents effective supervision in this situation?
    a. "Patient care can be frustrating at times. Mr. A has a hearing impairment, which probably adds to his confusion. It helps the hearing impaired if you face them directly when you speak and then speak slowly. Try demonstrating what you want him to do as you speak to him, if that makes sense for the situation. I'll come and check on you right after I administer this insulin."
    b. "It sounds like you need a break. Take a few minutes to calm down and then get back to Mr. A. He'll probably be done washing by the time you get back."
    c. "I know how you feel. Mr. A. can be very hard to work with. You should get the other aide to help you. Speak loudly into his left ear. That's his good ear."
    d. "You know, it really isn't right for nurses to get frustrated with patients who can't help the way they act. You're a better aide than that. Remember, Mr. A. is old and confused, and doesn't mean any harm. Go back in there and try again. Call me if you need help."

17. Mr. Kaufmann, a 77-year-old man with Alzheimer's disease, has become combative with the nursing staff. You assign a male UAP to his care. Choose the best answer from the following possible explanations about this delegation decision.
    a. It is a good delegation decision because the male UAP can handle a patient who is combative better than a female UAP can.
    b. It is not a good delegation decision because two UAPs will be needed to provide his care.
    c. It is a good delegation decision only if you make yourself available to help if the patient is confused.
    d. It is a good delegation decision only if the patient who is combative is in wrist restraints.

18. Which of the following questions represents the best approach to determining if a caregiver is experiencing burnout?
    a. "Are you tired of taking care of your husband/wife?"
    b. "Are you experiencing any personal health problems such as insomnia or fatigue?"
    c. "Have you ever felt like leaving your husband/wife?"
    d. "Do you feel you have too much to do in terms of caring for your husband/wife?"

19. Which organs of the body are primarily responsible for metabolizing and eliminating medications from the body?
    a. Gastrointestinal tract and kidneys
    b. Pancreas and lungs
    c. Liver and gastrointestinal tract
    d. Liver and kidneys

20. Many older patients experience a decline in renal function as they age. What effect does renal decline have on medications?
    a. Decline in renal function has very little effect on medications unless the patient goes into acute renal failure.
    b. Decline in renal function can cause excessive amounts of a drug to be left circulating in the blood.
    c. Decline in renal function can cause an increase in dilute urine elimination, thereby flushing out too much medication too quickly.
    d. Decline in renal function does not really affect medications because most drugs are rendered inactive by the liver.

21. Anticoagulant drugs (sometimes called "blood thinners") are broken down (metabolized) in the liver. Which of the following might be an outcome if a patient has undiagnosed liver disease but is started on anticoagulants?
    a. There will be an increase in bleeding tendencies.
    b. The drugs will be ineffective, leading to an increase in clotting tendencies.
    c. The drugs will be excreted from the body unchanged.
    d. The drugs will cause more harm to the liver, possibly leading to liver failure.

22. You are a home health nurse and one of your patients, Mrs. Cortes, has age-related macular degeneration and recently diagnosed type 2 diabetes. She speaks only a little English, and you cannot ascertain whether or not she knows how to take her medications because you do not speak Spanish. Which of the following represents the best intervention for addressing her educational need?
    a. Try to find a pharmacist in her neighborhood who speaks Spanish, can explain her medications to her, and will prepare the medication bottle labels in Spanish.
    b. Use a plastic weekly pill dispenser and fill it for her each week.
    c. Ask Mrs. Cortes who in her family can act as a translator and have that person present at the next visit, which is scheduled in 2 days. In the meantime, use a plastic pill dispenser and dispense her medications appropriately for the rest of today and the next.
    d. Try to reach a bilingual family member, but if that is not successful, teach her about the pills she should take by using universal symbols for daytime and nighttime or other symbols such as a clock that will indicate time of day.

23. Which of the following are teaching points to discuss with each patient regarding his or her medications?
    a. Reason for taking the medication
    b. Potential side effects and interactions
    c. How to store the medication
    d. When to take the medication

Part 3.   Review Questions

Fill in the blank with the correct age group by number (e.g., 65–75 years old). The definitions of the age group are general; there are no hard and fast definitions, and people of different ages may have characteristics of other age groups.

24. _____ people are usually retired, experiencing loss of spouses and same-age friends, may be exhibiting more physical changes, refraining from formerly enjoyable activities, and may be at greater risk for development of a psychosocial disorder such as depression.

25. _____ people are often in need of regular assistance because their health has declined significantly.

26. _____ people may have experienced a decline in physical status and are often still working.

27. _____ people are a group who has doubled in size over the past decade and a half. They are sometimes referred to as centenarians.

Choose the correct answer(s). In some questions, more than one answer is correct. Select all that apply.

28. Physical effects of aging result, over time, in a decline in performance. Which of the following influence the physical effects of aging?
    a. Lifestyle
    b. Genetics
    c. Chronic diseases
    d. Surgeries

29. The occurrence of cerebrovascular accidents (stroke) increase with age. What is one of the risk factors that a person can change on their own to decrease the risk for stroke?
    a. Irregular heart beat
    b. Hypertension
    c. Diet high in saturated fats
    d. Diabetes

30. An older person under your care who has been alert and oriented begins acting different than normal and appears to be hallucinating. Which of the following is the correct term for this?
    a. Depression
    b. Dementia
    c. Delirium
    d. Confusion

31. Which of the following is a common cause of dementia in older adults?
    a. Alzheimer's disease
    b. Diabetes
    c. Drug side effect
    d. Febrile state

32. An 89-year-old female has been admitted to the long-term care (LTC) facility where you work. She had tried to remain independent, but her arthritis now prevents her from ambulating in her home even with a walker, and her children felt she would be safer in an LTC facility. What neurological effects should you monitor for?
    a. Confusion
    b. Depression
    c. Delirium
    d. Dementia

33. Older adults may have decreased sensation. Which of the following is an important intervention aimed at preventing complications from this physiological change?
    a. Check the bath water to make sure it is hot enough.
    b. Check the bath water to make sure it is not too hot.
    c. Make sure the patient wears at least socks when ambulating.
    d. Tell the patient to clip toenails regularly.

34. Decreased renal function is associated with old age. Which of the following tests give information about renal function?
    a. Blood urea nitrogen (BUN), creatinine, and glomerular filtration rate (GFR)
    b. Blood urea nitrogen (BUN), white blood cell count, and hematocrit
    c. Blood urea nitrogen (BUN), creatinine, and white blood cell count
    d. Creatinine, hematocrit, and liver function tests (LFTs)

35. Older adults who have become incontinent are likely to feel very embarrassed about it. Which of the following comments best demonstrates the respect and care a nurse must show to avoid making the incontinent adult uncomfortable? Assume the patient is unable to change to dry clothes or pads independently but would be able to tell if she has voided.
    a. "I'm just checking to see if you're wet. Do you need a diaper change?"
    b. "Have you passed urine lately? I don't want you getting a rash!"
    c. "Hello, Mrs. Williams. Would you like to use the bathroom? It would be great if we can prevent one of those little accidents you have."
    d. "Hello, Mrs. Williams. I wanted to check to see if you needed to use the bathroom now or if you need help getting into fresh underwear."

36. Which of the following are interventions that address the issues of osteoporosis and the risk for broken bones?
    a. Make sure stairs are well lighted and that handrails are present.
    b. Suggest the patient lift light weights and wear ankle weights on his or her daily walk.
    c. Tell the patient which foods are high in potassium.
    d. Suggest the patient use an emergency help signaling device.

37. Which one of the following integumentary system changes puts the patient at greatest risk for complications from bedrest?
    a. Skin becomes thin and fragile
    b. Capillaries become fragile
    c. Decreased circulation to skin and underlying tissue
    d. Tendency to bruise easily

38. Which of the following interventions will help prevent pressure sores for the patient with impaired mobility?
    a. Provide skin care several times per day if the patient is on bedrest.
    b. Place pillows between knees and ankles when in side-lying positions.
    c. Assess pressure points for erythema at least every 4 hours, sometimes as often as every 2 hours.
    d. Encourage adequate fluids and nutrition, and provide protein supplements if needed.

39. Which of the following signs or symptoms suggest significant changes in cardiovascular health?
    a. Shortness of breath with exertion
    b. Heart rate of 100 beats per minute
    c. Bilateral ankle swelling
    d. Capillary refill of 5 seconds

40. Older adults often have trouble with constipation. What is the physiological reason for constipation that is associated with old age?
   a. Changes in appetite
   b. Decreased peristalsis
   c. Insufficient fiber in the diet
   d. Using supplements such as Ensure

41. Older adults may not empty their bladders completely when they void because of changes in neuromuscular functioning of the bladder muscle or, in men, enlargement of the prostate gland. Which of the following is a common complication of insufficient bladder emptying?
   a. Constipation from enlarged bladder pressing on lower gastrointestinal tract
   b. Renal failure
   c. Urinary tract infection
   d. Bladder spasms

42. Older adults may experience a decline in sexual desire as they age. This may be related to which of the following?
   a. Erectile dysfunction
   b. Menopause
   c. Changes in hormone production
   d. Natural result of aging

43. You care for a resident in a long-term facility. She receives a phone call informing her that her older sister has died. Which of the following interventions will be most helpful for her at this time?
   a. Give her the number of a support group.
   b. Contact the facility's chaplain.
   c. Sit quietly with her.
   d. Tell her that grieving is a process with several stages.

44. A 72-year-old patient is brought to the doctor's office by his son for a checkup. As you are helping him disrobe, you notice several bruises on his stomach. You ask him if he has fallen and he says no, he got them leaning over the sink doing dishes. Which of the following represents your next action?
   a. Suggest he pad the edge of the countertop with foam rubber.
   b. Gently suggest that it is okay to tell you that he fell—that it does not mean he will be put in a nursing home.
   c. Ask him if he is taking anticoagulants or if he has been in the hospital recently.
   d. Ask him about his relationship with his son.

45. Which of the following concepts is(are) important to remember when you work in a long-term care facility?
   a. The residents are still sick, even if they are not in an acute care facility.
   b. Many residents would prefer to be left alone, and you should honor their wishes.
   c. The people consider their rooms their personal residences.
   d. Residents should be encouraged to wear pajama-type clothing for comfort.

46. Fall prevention is an extremely important consideration when caring for older adults. Which of the following are interventions you can perform that will help prevent falls?
   a. Get the help of coworkers when transferring a patient with impaired mobility.
   b. Make sure the patient or resident is wearing shoes with nonskid soles.
   c. Keep walkways clear of small articles, electrical cords, and throw rugs.
   d. Never leave a resident who uses a walker while he or she is ambulating.

Write a brief answer to the following questions.

47. List three important measures to take while assisting a resident with bathing and hygiene in a shared bathroom at a long-term care facility. Provide a rationale for each intervention.

_____

_____

_____

_____

_____

_____

48. List several nursing responsibilities related to providing meals to residents in long-term care facilities.

_____

_____

_____

_____

_____

_____

49. List at least three important interventions that must be performed for the resident who is incontinent. Explain why the intervention is important.

_____

_____

_____

_____

_____

50. List several interventions that are required when caring for patients/residents with impaired mobility.

_____

_____

_____

_____

_____

Indicate whether the following statements are True (T) or False (F).

51. _____ In general, a head-to-toe assessment of residents in a long-term care facility should be performed once a day.

52. _____ In general, vital signs of long-term care residents should be assessed once a week or once a month, depending on the facility's policy.

53. _____ Unless indicated by unexpected events, documentation in a long-term care facility is usually done once per week.

54. _____ Polypharmacy refers to the ingestion of many different medications.

55. _____ One reason polypharmacy occurs is because an older individual has several different physicians prescribing medications for him or her and each is unaware of what the other has prescribed.

56. _____ Polypharmacy greatly increases the risk for drug interactions.

57. _____ Patients' lack of knowledge about the medications they take is a factor in polypharmacy.

58. _____ As a nurse, you can review each medication to assess for its purpose and for overlap among drugs.

Part 4. Application and Critical Thinking Questions

Write a brief answer to the following questions.

59. Older adults frequently have cardiovascular problems. Based on the discussion of changes in cardiovascular functioning provided in this chapter, list signs and symptoms you might expect to see if the older adult is experiencing a cardiovascular problem. Explain why these might be occurring.

_____

_____

_____

_____

_____

_____

60. You work in a long-term care facility and note that the residents seem bored. What are some actions you can take to alleviate their boredom? Consider how different activities may address other issues besides boredom. (Hint: Begin a group exercise program for residents in wheelchairs.)

61. List and explain what you would assess when you notice a resident's appetite has declined.

_____

_____

_____

_____

_____

62. Describe assessment findings or patient behaviors that would lead you to suspect the older adult is being abused.

_____

_____

_____

_____

_____

63. Describe some of the positive aspects of aging. Explain some ways that nurses might interact inappropriately with older patients or residents and what they should do instead.

_____

_____

_____

_____

_____

Documentation Exercise

▶ *Scenario:*

It is April 12, 2017. You are caring for a patient who was hospitalized with elevated blood sugar and side effects from medications. Mr. Donald Baxter is a 71-year-old man with mild cognitive impairment, heart disease, and diabetes. His date of birth is 4/19/1945. His hospital identification number is 13572. He is in Room 409. He was attempting to manage his own medications prior to hospitalization. His wife is in ill health and had not realized that he was not taking his medications correctly.

At 2 p.m. you begin patient teaching. You instruct the patient and his wife regarding the medications he is to take. He must take a heart pill, a diuretic, and a diabetes pill every morning. At noon he is to take a potassium supplement. At suppertime he will be taking another diabetes pill and a medication to relieve leg pain during the night. Many of his pills are small, white, and round, so he gets them confused easily. He and his wife explain that he has difficulty remembering to take the diabetes pill with supper and the potassium supplement at noon.

You assist the patient and his wife in setting up a pill box with a week's supply of medications prepared. At 2:45 p.m. you contact the prescribing physician, Dr. Holsted, and obtain permission for Mr. Baxter to take the potassium supplement in the morning with his other medications, emphasizing that he is to eat breakfast so that he does not take it on an empty stomach. You also obtain permission for him to take the medication for nighttime leg pain at supper with his second diabetes medication. This decreases his frequency of taking medications from four times per day to two times per day, which is more manageable for him.

You return to patient teaching at 3:10 p.m. You explain what each pill is for and what to watch for in terms of side effects or adverse effects. After several attempts, Mr. Baxter is able to tell you what each pill is for and when he should take each one. His wife is able to tell you the kinds of adverse effects she will watch for and then call the doctor to report. Both the patient and his wife thank you for helping them get his medication schedule more manageable for them.

64. Document your patient teaching on the nurse's note form (Fig. 32-1).

		Mission Regional Hospital
Patient _____		
ID# _____ RM _____		
BD _____-_____-_____		
Admit _____-_____-_____		
Physician _____		

Date	Time	Nurse's Notes

Figure 32.1 Nurse's note.

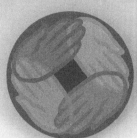

Care of the Surgical Patient

Name:	
Date:	
Course:	
Instructor:	

Part 1. Key Terms Review

Match the following Key Term(s) or italicized words from your text with the correct description.

_____ 1. Anesthesia

_____ 2. Bier block

_____ 3. Cosmetic

_____ 4. Exploratory

_____ 5. Corrective

_____ 6. Palliative

_____ 7. Local anesthesia

_____ 8. Regional anesthesia

_____ 9. Epidural anesthesia

_____10. Conscious sedation

_____11. General anesthesia

a. Surgery done to provide further data and determine a diagnosis for a problem

b. Surgery done to repair an anatomical or congenital defect

c. Surgery to alleviate symptoms and provide comfort but does not necessarily cure the disease or heal the injury

d. Surgery performed to change or improve one's physical appearance

e. A very small area of tissue is blocked from sensory perception by injection of a local anesthetic numbing agent such as lidocaine or Novocain

f. A small catheter inserted into the epidural space of the spinal column to provide a continual administration of a stronger anesthesia agent

g. The loss of sensation with or without loss of consciousness accomplished by the administration of inhaled or injected medications

h. Specific nerves and the region innervated by the nerves, such as a finger, or larger areas of the body, such as an arm or lower half of the body, are blocked from sensory perception by injection of a local anesthetic numbing agent such as lidocaine or Novocain

i. Techniques used to isolate the administration of local anesthetic to a specific nerve or region to prevent transmission of sensory information to and from that part of the body; numbness or loss of feeling and loss of ability to voluntarily move the area

j. The patient is totally unconscious

k. The patient is asleep but not totally unconscious

Fill in the blank with the correct Key Term(s) or italicized words from your text.

12. Insertion of an endotracheal tube into the patient's trachea to maintain an open airway and administer inhalant anesthesia and oxygen is _____.

13. Removal of an endotracheal tube is known as _____.

14. _____ surgery uses a specialized scope and instruments in place of making a large incision.

15. A rapid and severe rise in body temperature that occurs while under a general anesthesia as a result of an inherited genetic trait is called _____.

16. How well the edges of the surgical incision meet and align with one another is called _____.

17. Another name for a recovery room is _____.

18. When the wound edges separate it is known as _____.

19. _____ are stockings applied to the legs to assist return of venous blood back to the right side of the heart.

20. _____ are wrapped around the legs to assist the return of venous blood back to the right side of the heart.

Part 2. Connection Questions

Choose the correct answer(s). In some questions, more than one answer is correct. Select all that apply.

21. Kelly Majetic is going to have a face-lift surgery tomorrow. You know that this is what type of surgery?
    a. Corrective
    b. Cosmetic
    c. Palliative
    d. Exploratory
    e. Curative

22. Marla Monett is scheduled to have breast enlargement surgery today at 0830. This surgery is classified as what type of surgery?
    a. Corrective
    b. Cosmetic
    c. Palliative
    d. Exploratory
    e. Curative

23. You are caring for Allen Julius, who has been diagnosed with advanced cancer of the liver. He has been suffering severe discomfort as a result of ascites, the collection of fluid within the peritoneal cavity that puts pressure on all the abdominal organs. The patient and physician have decided that the best course of treatment is palliative: to relieve the discomfort by surgically placing a peritoneal drainage tube to drain the excess fluid. His wife asks you if this surgery will cure him. Your best response would be:
    a. "This procedure is not curative, but it will help to provide him with a higher quality of life by relieving the discomfort of the fluid that has been collecting in the peritoneal cavity."
    b. "Yes, removing the fluid would cure your husband."
    c. "No, of course not."
    d. "You do not really think we can cure your husband at this late stage in the disease process, do you? We have to be realistic."

24. Margaret Gruntmeir has been complaining of abdominal pain for several weeks, and tests have proved inconclusive. The physician has explained to Ms. Gruntmeir that she feels the best course of action is to open the abdomen surgically and see what might be causing the problem. You know that this type of surgical procedure would be considered to be:
    a. Corrective
    b. Cosmetic
    c. Palliative
    d. Exploratory
    e. Curative

Classify the following surgeries for purpose and degree of urgency.

25. _____ Reconstruction of severed ligament in the knee

26. _____ Tummy tuck

27. _____ Cholecystectomy (removal of the gallbladder)

28. _____ Colectomy (removal of cancerous portion of the colon)

29. _____ CABG (coronary artery bypass graft after a severe heart attack)

30. _____ Mastectomy (removal of cancerous breast)

31. _____ Breast biopsy

32. _____ Nerve block to relieve pain

33. _____ Placement of a venous access device for administration of analgesia

a. Corrective
b. Cosmetic
c. Palliative
d. Exploratory
e. Curative

Choose the correct answer(s). In some questions, more than one answer is correct. Select all that apply.

34. There are several advantages to having laparoscopic surgery rather than the traditional opening of the operative area with a large incision. Which of the following is not an advantage?
    a. Reduction in risk for infection
    b. Less postoperative pain
    c. Easier-to-perform procedure
    d. Shorter recovery time

35. Research shows that patients who receive preoperative teaching do better after surgery. Which of the following are benefits of preoperative teaching?
    a. Reduction in anxiety and fear
    b. Reduction in complications
    c. Smoother, shorter recovery
    d. Better chance of optimal healing

Part 3. Review Questions

Choose the correct answer(s). In some questions, more than one answer is correct. Select all that apply.

36. Pain control is one of the biggest issues for the patient postoperatively. Which of the following is(are) accurate?
    a. The patient heals better and faster if there is less use of pain medications.
    b. It is easy to become addicted to narcotic analgesic medications if the patient uses the medication too often.
    c. It is important to ensure that the patient understands that there are medications that should be taken for pain control.
    d. It is easier to control pain if the patient asks for medication before the pain gets too severe.

37. Which of the following is(are) a reason(s) to use SCDs and TED?
    a. Decrease risk for pneumonia
    b. Decrease risk for deep vein thrombosis
    c. Prevent pooling of blood in the legs
    d. Aid in venous blood return
    e. Reduce the need to ambulate a patient when you are busy

38. There are various purposes for which preoperative medications may be given. Which of the following purposes serve as a legitimate reason to administer a preoperative medication?
    a. Provide relief of apprehension and anxiety
    b. Provide sedation
    c. Shorten surgery time
    d. Reduce risk for pneumonia
    e. Decrease gastric volume and acidity
    f. Prevent nausea and vomiting
    g. Dry secretions and prevent aspiration

39. Who has the responsibility to obtain consent for surgery?
    a. The nurse
    b. Office personnel
    c. The surgeon
    d. The unit clerk

40. Which member of the surgical team is the primary patient advocate?
    a. The scrub nurse
    b. The surgeon
    c. The anesthesiologist
    d. The circulating nurse
    e. The assistant surgeon
    f. The certified registered nurse anesthetist (CRNA)

41. Why is it a good idea to call a *time-out* prior to initiating surgery?
    a. Helps to reduce performance of surgery on the wrong side or limb
    b. Helps to ensure the correct patient
    c. Ensures that the correct procedure is about to be performed
    d. To confirm that the physician really needs to perform the surgical procedure
    e. Ensures that the surgical consent has been signed

42. A patient must be intubated for which type of anesthesia?
    a. Local anesthesia
    b. Regional anesthesia
    c. Conscious sedation
    d. General anesthesia

43. Who is responsible for ensuring that a postoperative patient's vital signs are stable after the patient has returned to his or her room?
    a. The CNA
    b. The UAP
    c. The licensed nurse assigned to the patient
    d. The surgeon

Part 4. Application and Critical Thinking Questions

Write a brief answer to the following questions.

44. A patient has just returned to her room from PACU after a general anesthesia and gastric bypass. How often should her vital signs be taken over the next 24 hours?

_____

_____

_____

_____

_____

45. Which two organs are responsible for metabolism of anesthesia?

_____

_____

46. List at least three laboratory tests that provide you with information about a patient's nutritional status.

_____

_____

▶ *Situation:* Question 47 refers to this scenario.

Andrea Wilson is scheduled for an elective surgery, which is canceled on review of her preoperative laboratory white blood cell count. It is very low at 1,700/mm³.

47. When she asks what this test result means, how do you explain to her what it means?

_____

_____

▶ *Situation:* Question 48 refers to this scenario.

Tracy Pugh was scheduled last month to have an elective cosmetic surgical procedure done tomorrow. Her preoperative laboratory results have just been posted. Her platelet count, at 750,000/mm³, is too low to proceed with surgery.

48. Her low platelet count puts Tracy at risk for what complication?

_____

49. Before an elective surgery is performed on a 24-year-old female patient, which additional laboratory test might be ordered that would not be ordered on a male patient of the same age?

_____

50. What types of information should be included in preoperative teaching? List a minimum of eight items.

_____

_____

_____

_____

_____

51. Which member of the surgical team must be a registered nurse as opposed to being a licensed practical nurse? _____

Documentation Exercise

▸ *Scenario:*

You have been assigned to Terri Kirby, the preoperative patient in Room 617 who was admitted on 4/7/17. Her ID is #987123 and her birth date is 10/1/88. She is scheduled for surgery with a general anesthesia later tomorrow. You have just performed the first portion of your preoperative teaching, which included leg exercises and turning, coughing, and deep breathing techniques. The patient was able to demonstrate correctly how to perform them. She also acknowledged to you verbally that she understood the importance of performing these tasks after surgery tomorrow. The current date is 4/8/17 and it is 1015.

52. Use a blank nurse's note form (Fig. 33-1) and narrative documentation to chart this teaching session. Use appropriate abbreviations and be succinct. Include both the implementation and evaluation phases of the teaching.

Patient _____		Mission Regional Hospital
ID# _____ RM _____		
BD _____-_____-_____		
Admit _____-_____-_____		
Physician _____		

Date	Time	Nurse's Notes

Figure 33.1 Nurse's note.

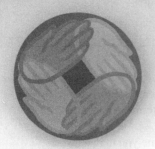

Phlebotomy and Blood Specimens

Name:	
Date:	
Course:	
Instructor:	

Part 1. Key Terms Review

Match the following Key Term(s) or italicized words from your text with the correct description.

_____ 1. Petechiae

_____ 2. Septicemia

_____ 3. Syncope

_____ 4. Anaerobic

_____ 5. Hemolysis

_____ 6. Anastomoses

_____ 7. Tourniquet

_____ 8. Sclerosed

_____ 9. Hematoma

_____ 10. Lymphostasis

_____ 11. Aerobic

_____ 12. Evacuated tube or
Vacutainer tube

_____ 13. Tortuous

_____ 14. Blood culture

_____ 15. Hemoconcentration

a. Organisms that can live and replicate without oxygen

b. Organisms that grow and replicate in the presence of oxygen

c. Junctions where veins join other veins and arteries join arteries

d. Glass tube closed with a colored rubber stopper from which air has been evacuated, used to draw blood specimens

e. Fainting

f. Destruction of red blood cells

g. Once a lymph node is removed, lymph fluid does not move and remains static

h. Pinpoint areas of hemorrhage

i. Veins that have many twists and turns

j. Veins that feel hard and ropey

k. Bruise

l. A concentration of red blood cells in the blood sample resulting from a decrease in the volume of plasma allowed to flow

m. Blood specimen drawn to determine if organisms are present in the blood, and if so, which specific organism is the culprit

n. Infection of one's blood

o. A rubber strap that can be snugly wrapped around the arm to occlude the venous return of blood toward the heart

Part 2. Connection Questions

Choose the correct answer(s). In some questions, more than one answer is correct. Select all that apply.

16. Why is it important that you tell the patient exactly what you are about to do before you begin?
    a. To gain the patient's cooperation
    b. To delay the start of the task
    c. To reduce patient anxiety
    d. To demonstrate your knowledge

17. Which of the following statements is(are) accurate regarding veins?
    a. Veins are deeper than arteries.
    b. Veins carry deoxygenated blood.
    c. Veins carry blood back to the heart.
    d. Vein walls are thicker than arterial walls.

18. Which one of the following statements is not accurate when describing veins and arteries?
    a. Veins have valves; arteries do not.
    b. Valves control the direction of blood flow in veins.
    c. Arteries have higher blood pressure than veins.
    d. Veins have thicker walls than arteries.
    e. Veins must fight against gravity to return blood to the heart.

19. The vein of choice for phlebotomy is:
    a. The median cubital
    b. The basilic
    c. The cephalic
    d. Any vein that is not tortuous

20. Which of the following is most important when assessing for a suitable vein to use for venipuncture?
    a. Your vision
    b. Your sense of touch
    c. Whether the patient is left- or right-handed
    d. Whether the vein is deep or shallow

21. There are several tips you may use to find a suitable vein for venipuncture. Which of the following techniques should not be used?
    a. Have the patient hang the proposed arm dependently to allow blood to better fill the veins of the arm.
    b. Use an alcohol swab to apply rubbing friction in an attempt to stimulate the vein to distend.
    c. Using your fingers, slap the skin over the vein in an attempt to stimulate the vein to distend.
    d. Apply a warm pack to the site for 5 to 10 minutes to dilate the vein.

22. Some of the following statements are true regarding the correct techniques for phlebotomy. Which statement(s) is(are) true?
    a. The maximum length of time you may leave a tourniquet in place on the patient's arm is 3 minutes.
    b. The tourniquet should be applied 6 to 8 inches above the proposed puncture site.
    c. The labels should be applied to the tubes prior to filling them with blood.
    d. If the patient's skin is fragile, you should apply the tourniquet over the gown sleeve to prevent skin tears.

23. The labels you apply to the blood specimen tubes should contain some of the following data. Which data should not be included on the label?
    a. Patient's first and last name
    b. Hospital identification number
    c. Room number
    d. Physician's name
    e. Type of test ordered
    f. Date test was ordered
    g. Date specimen was collected
    h. Time specimen was collected
    i. Patient's initials
    j. Your initials

24. You should avoid which of the following actions that can cause hemolysis?
    a. Using a 20- or 22-gauge needle and syringe
    b. Leaving the tourniquet on longer than 1 minute
    c. Using an evacuated tube set and a 25-gauge needle
    d. Withdrawing the blood slowly when using a needle and syringe

25. What action(s) will help to protect you from bloodborne pathogens during phlebotomy?
    a. Washing your hands prior to the procedure
    b. Washing your hands after the procedure
    c. Wearing gloves during the procedure
    d. Activating the needle safety device immediately after removing your gloves

Part 3. Application and Critical Thinking Questions

Choose the correct answer(s). In some questions, more than one answer is correct. Select all that apply.

▶ *Scenario: Questions 26 through 28 refer to the following scenario.*

You are preparing to draw blood specimens from an adult man who weighs approximately 190 pounds and has good veins. You are to draw blood for cultures, glucose, complete blood cell count, and electrolytes. You have decided to use the Vacutainer evacuated tube system.

26. You are preparing to draw the blood specimen and know that you must protect yourself against bloodborne pathogens. How will you accomplish this?
    a. Scrub the intended site with alcohol.
    b. Monitor the patient's chart for a history of blood-borne pathogens.
    c. Wash your hands prior to drawing blood.
    d. Apply clean examination gloves.

Write a brief answer to the following questions.

29. When performing skin punctures, what sites are commonly used in an infant, older child, and adult?

_____

_____

_____

30. You are performing phlebotomy on an elderly patient using a needle and syringe setup. Besides hemolysis, what can happen if you pull the plunger back too rapidly?

_____

_____

_____

_____

_____

_____

31. Explain the purpose of applying a tourniquet for phlebotomy.

_____

_____

_____

27. What color tubes will you need for these tests?
    a. Red
    b. Gray
    c. Light blue
    d. Yellow
    e. Lavender
    f. Green

28. In what sequence will you draw the colored tubes?
    (1) _____ (2) _____
    (3) _____ (4) _____

32. Briefly explain why you should not draw blood from the arm on the same side the patient has had a mastectomy.

_____

_____

_____

33. If you are drawing both aerobic and anaerobic blood cultures using the long-necked specimen bottles, which one will you draw first? _____

34. List the eight colored tube tops in the correct order of draw according to the text.
    (1) _____ (2) _____ (3) _____ (4) _____
    (5) _____ (6) _____ (7) _____ (8) _____

Documentation Exercise

▶ *Scenario:*

You have just drawn blood specimens (with a single stick) for electrolytes, complete blood cell count (CBC), and a basic metabolic panel (BMP) at the left antecubital fossa from the median cubital vein. The patient's name is Turbi Kurbo, and she is in Room 617. Her hospital ID is #987123. Her birthdate is 10/1/88. Today's date is 4/8/17, and the current time is 1315.

35. On a nurse's note (Fig. 34-1), document the phlebotomy that you just performed. Use the appropriate abbreviations, and include your signature and credentials.

Patient _____		
ID# _____ RM _____		Mission Regional Hospital
BD _____-_____-_____		
Admit _____-_____-_____		
Physician _____		

Date	Time	Nurse's Notes

Figure 34.1 Nurse's note.

Medication Administration

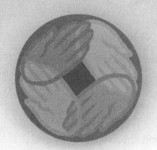

Researching and Preparing Medications

Name: _____

Date: _____

Course: _____

Instructor: _____

Part 1. Key Terms Review

Match the following Key Term(s) or italicized words from your text with the correct description.

_____ 1. Brand name

_____ 2. Topical route

_____ 3. Side effect

_____ 4. Therapeutic level

_____ 5. Chemical name

_____ 6. Oral route

_____ 7. Toxicity

_____ 8. Desired effect

_____ 9. Over-the-counter (OTC) medications

a. The exact ingredients of a medication

b. Route by which medications are taken through the mouth

c. Medicines available without a prescription

d. The short, easy-to-remember name of a drug

e. The reason a medication is prescribed

f. The route by which medicines are applied to the skin

g. Occurs when an unintended outcome of a medication takes place

h. Amount of medicine in the blood necessary to cause the desired effects on target organs

i. Too much of a medication in the body

Fill in the blank with the correct Key Term(s) or italicized words from your text.

10. A shorthand version of a drug's chemical name assigned by the U.S. Adopted Name Council (USANC) is known as the _____.

11. _____ are available with a written direction from a health-care provider with prescriptive authority.

12. All medications given beneath the skin are administered via the _____.

13. When medications are applied through the rectum, vagina, eye, or ear or are inhaled into the lungs, they are given by the _____.

14. Unintended effects that are more severe or harmful than side effects are called _____.

15. _____ occurs when the patient's body reacts to a medication as a foreign invader to be destroyed.

16. A comprehensive book that contains detailed information about a large number of medications, containing the same information as the drug package inserts, is called the _____.

17. A drug reference book designed specifically for nurses is called a _____.

18. The document that lists the patient's medications and the times they are to be given, on which the nurse initials administration of the drugs, is the _____.

Part 2. Connection Questions

Choose the correct answer(s). In some questions, more than one answer is correct. Select all that apply.

19. You are preparing to give medications to your assigned patient in clinical. The orders are for eight different medications, a nitroglycerin patch, and an insulin injection. What will your instructor expect you to know about these medications before you administer them?
    a. The classification of each medication
    b. The desired effect of each medication
    c. The major side effects of each medication
    d. The name of the physician who ordered each medication
    e. Laboratory values to be checked before giving any of the medications
    f. Vital signs to be checked before giving any of the medications

20. What factors can contribute to the risk for a nurse to develop a drug abuse problem?
    a. Nurses deal with high work-related stress.
    b. Nurses are statistically more at risk for drug abuse.
    c. Nurses have easy access to drugs.
    d. Nurses are less likely to be held accountable for missing drugs.

21. What would happen if a nurse was caught diverting drugs?
    a. Very little would happen because it would be difficult to prove or get a conviction.
    b. The situation would be dealt with by the nursing supervisor and hospital administration.
    c. The nurse could face arrest and criminal charges.
    d. The nurse would be referred to a program where he or she could get help.

22. You are administering medications to your assigned patients. Just as you enter a female patient's room with the prepared medicines in a cup, the patient enters the bathroom for a shower. You then get an urgent call to another patient's room. What will you do?
    a. Ask the CNA who is assisting the patient with a shower to give her the medicines after the shower.
    b. Ask the CNA who is assisting the patient with a shower to give her the medicines immediately.
    c. Tell another nurse to respond to the urgent call because you have to wait to give this patient's medicines to her after she gets out of the shower.
    d. Interrupt the patient's shower preparations long enough to give her the medications and ensure that she has swallowed them.

23. You are administering medication to a child. How can you ensure that you have calculated the correct dose before you administer it?
    a. Call a pharmacist and ask for the ranges for pediatric dosages of this medication.
    b. Ask another nurse to check your calculations and verify that it is the correct dose.
    c. Ask the child's parent how much of the medicine has been administered to the child in the past.
    d. Determine half of the adult dose and administer that amount to the child.

24. Why are elderly patients at greater risk for development of drug toxicity?
    a. Impaired liver and kidney function, causing the drug to build up in the blood
    b. Impaired ability to see and take the correct dosage
    c. Impaired ability of the stomach and intestines to absorb the correct amount of the drug
    d. Aging causes slowed metabolism, which leads to drug toxicity

25. You are caring for a patient taking digoxin for congestive heart failure. During your shift, the patient complains of nausea. What will you do before giving his next dose of digoxin?
    a. Call the physician and get an order for an antiemetic to give with the digoxin.
    b. Give an antacid 30 minutes before giving the digoxin to prevent stomach irritation.
    c. Check the patient's digoxin level on the chart to determine that it is not elevated.
    d. Ask the patient if he thinks the medicine is making him feel nauseated.

26. Your patient is taking Lasix 40 mg PO as a diuretic. When you checked, the patient's potassium level was low, at 3.3. You held the Lasix and notified the PA with the laboratory results. The PA then said to give the Lasix and also ordered a potassium supplement, K-tab, 20 mg to be given to this patient bid. How does this order resolve your concern?
    a. The potassium supplement will replace the potassium that is being removed by the Lasix.
    b. It does not resolve the problem, and you will need to talk to your supervisor about the orders.
    c. The Lasix will work more effectively when there is more potassium in the patient's blood.
    d. Both the Lasix and the K-tab will help restore the patient's potassium level to the normal range.

Part 3. Review Questions

Choose the correct answer(s). In some questions, more than one answer is correct. Select all that apply.

27. The trade name of a drug is also referred to as the:
    a. Brand name
    b. Chemical name
    c. Proprietary name
    d. Generic name

28. A pharmaceutical company has developed a new medicine that was costly to create. How will the company be compensated for the cost of their research and development?
    a. They will set the price of the medication very high to allow rebates from insurance companies.
    b. They will be awarded money from the government for developing a new medicine.
    c. They will get a portion of the payments that other companies receive when they sell the drug.
    d. They will be allowed to sell the medication with no competition for approximately 10 years.

29. Which of the following is an example of an over-the-counter medication?
    a. Hydrocodone (Lortab)
    b. Amoxicillin (Amoxil)
    c. Acetaminophen (Tylenol)
    d. Cefazolin (Ancef)

30. The oral route of medication administration includes:
    a. Sublingual and buccal medicines
    b. Inhalants and mists
    c. Ointments and patches
    d. Eye and ear drops

31. Schedule II drugs:
    a. Have a high potential for abuse
    b. Must be counted and accounted for
    c. Have no medicinal purpose
    d. Include morphine, codeine, oxycodone, and meperidine
    e. Must be kept under double lock

32. Which patient is most likely to have a drug reaction?
    a. A patient with kidney failure who is on dialysis
    b. A patient who is more physically active than the average person
    c. A patient with no known drug allergies (NKDA)
    d. A patient who has never had a reaction to a medicine in the past

33. A 46-year-old female patient developed swelling of the tongue and throat after taking a new antibiotic. She went to the ER because she was having difficulty breathing. Which drug effect has occurred?
    a. A desired effect
    b. A side effect
    c. An adverse effect
    d. A severe adverse effect

34. A patient with pneumonia is allergic to cephalosporin antibiotics. He tells you that he breaks out in a rash and itches if he takes it. The physician has prescribed Cefazolin (Ancef) for him because it is one of the few antibiotics that will kill the bacteria cultured from his sputum. What will you do?
    a. Hold the medication and notify the physician.
    b. Give the medication and administer oral diphenhydramine (Benadryl) without an order because it is an OTC medication.
    c. Ask the supervising nurse to give the medication because the patient may have an allergic reaction.
    d. Give the medication and watch the patient closely for any signs of anaphylaxis.

35. You are caring for a patient who has an order for an IV antibiotic. When you hang the second bag, the patient goes into an anaphylactic reaction. Which actions will you expect to perform?
    a. Stop the medication immediately.
    b. Slow the IV rate and administer diphenhydramine (Benadryl) via the IV route.
    c. Follow the facility policy for responding to anaphylaxis.
    d. Increase IV fluids to help increase the blood pressure.
    e. Obtain IV epinephrine in case it is needed.

36. You are caring for a patient who is taking valproic acid (Depakote) to prevent seizure activity. The therapeutic blood level of this medication is 50 to 100 g/mL. The patient's laboratory results show a level of 108 g/mL. The medication is ordered to be administered orally at 0900. You are caring for this patient and it is 0800. What will you do?
    a. Give the medication as ordered; the blood level is only slightly elevated and the physician will see it when making rounds later.
    b. Hold the medication until the physician sees the patient next; then you can ask whether to continue giving the medication.
    c. Give the medication as ordered; administer one aspirin with it to bind some of the drug.
    d. Hold the medication; notify the physician of the blood level and obtain orders regarding the administration of the medication.

37. The patient you are caring for has been placed on warfarin (Coumadin) to prevent blood clots. Which teaching will you provide?
    a. Do not take aspirin or products containing aspirin while you are taking Coumadin.
    b. Report excessive bruising or bleeding from the gums, eyes, kidneys, intestines, or vagina.
    c. Do not consume milk or other dairy products while you are taking Coumadin.
    d. Do not drink grapefruit juice or eat grapefruit while you are taking Coumadin.

38. Which is true of the PDR?
    a. It contains only one index, so you must know the generic name of a drug to look it up.
    b. It is written specifically for nurses and includes topics for patient teaching.
    c. It contains colored pictures of many drugs in the Product Identification Section.
    d. It contains medication chemical composition, indications for use, contraindications, warnings, routes, and administration guidelines.

39. Before administering any antihypertensive medication, you will first:
    a. Ask the patient if he or she is allergic to any antibiotics.
    b. Check the chart for the most recent temperature readings.
    c. Ensure that any ordered blood cultures have already been drawn.
    d. Check the patient's blood pressure to ensure that it is not too low.

Fill in the blank.

40. List the six rights of medication administration.

    a. Right _____

    b. Right _____

    c. Right _____

    d. Right _____

    e. Right _____

    f. Right _____

41. Identify the three times to check the medication, dose, route, and patient to ensure that you are administering the medication safely.

    a. _____

    b. _____

    c. _____

Write a brief answer to the following questions.

42. If a patient is taking numerous medications, how can you be sure that you have them all when you are preparing them?

_____

_____

_____

43. A patient is taking simvastatin (Lipitor) for high cholesterol levels. What patient teaching will you provide regarding interaction of this medication with foods, beverages, and supplements?

_____

_____

_____

44. The following medication order appears in your patient's chart:

2-13-17. 1400. Amiodarone hydrochloride 200 mg PO.

R. Burton, MD

What is missing from this order? _____

What will you do before administering this medication?

_____

_____

_____

_____

45. What will you check before administering antiarrhythmic medications to your patients?

_____

46. Under what circumstances would you hold these medications?

_____

_____

_____

47. What are signs that a patient is receiving too much of an anticoagulant medication?

_____

_____

_____

_____

48. Which vital sign will you check before administering vasodilators to your patients?

_____

49. What assessment will you make before administering laxatives and stool softeners to your patients?

_____

_____

_____

_____

50. What assessment will you make before administering antidiabetic medications?

_____

51. What signs will you check for before administering anti-inflammatory medications?

_____

_____

_____

_____

52. What is the purpose of tall man letters in drug names?

_____

_____

_____

Part 4. Application and Critical Thinking Questions

For these drug dosage calculations, use the formula in your book or another formula provided by your instructor to find the correct dosages to administer. Show all of the calculation steps, not just the answer.

53. Physician's order: *pravastatin sodium (Pravachol) 20 mg PO daily at bedtime.*
    Drug on hand: *Pravachol 40-mg oral tablets*
    Safety: Prior to giving, assess drug allergies.
    How many tablets will you administer per dose?

    _____

54. Physician's order: *aspirin 600 mg PO every 4–6 hours prn*
    Fever above 102°F.
    Drug on hand: *aspirin 5-gr tablets*
    Safety: Prior to administering, remember to assess the time interval since the last dose. Also assess drug allergies.
    How many tablets will you administer per dose?

    _____

55. Physician's order: *warfarin (Coumadin) 6 mg PO daily at noon.*
    Drug on hand: *warfarin 2-mg oral tablets*
    Safety: Prior to administering, you must assess the patient's most current PT/INR (prothrombin time/international ratio) laboratory results to ensure that it is safe to give the warfarin. Also assess drug allergies.
    How many tablets will you administer per dose?

    _____

56. Physician's order: *atenolol (Tenormin) 75 mg PO daily in the early morning.*
    Drug on hand: *Two (2) different strength tablets are available.*
    atenolol 25-mg tablets
    atenolol 50-mg tablets
    Safety: Prior to giving, assess drug allergies. Monitor BP.
    Can you use any of these strength tablets? _____
    How many tablets will you administer per dose if you use the 25-mg tablets? _____
    How many tablets will you administer per dose if you use the 50-mg tablets? _____

57. Physician's order: *potassium gluconate elixir (Kaon) 50 mEq PO bid*
    Drug on hand: *Kaon Elixir 20 mEq/5 mL*
    How many milliliters will you administer per dose?

    _____

    Safety: Prior to giving, assess drug allergies. Also assess the patient's current serum K+ level.

Write a brief answer to the following question.

▶ *Scenario:*

You are preparing to give medications to your patient. She has 10 oral medications due at 0900 plus eye drops. You have verified the physician's orders with the MAR. There is one medication you do not recognize, and you have looked it up. As you begin to prepare the medication, you are interrupted twice by other staff members with questions. You feel like you are scattered rather than focused as you begin preparing the medications. You notice that one of her medications is not provided in the exact unit of measurement that it is ordered. Your patient is receiving two blood pressure medications and a cardiac glycoside.

58. Determine what steps you need to take to prepare these medications and the order in which you will perform them.

_____

_____

_____

_____

_____

_____

Documentation Exercise

Today is April 24, 2017. You are administering medications to Ms. Ebonie Washington, a 51-year-old patient with a diagnosis of coronary artery disease and hypertension who was admitted on April 22, 2017. She is in Room 409 and her hospital ID is #4982376. Her date of birth is February 7, 1966. At 9 a.m. you give Ms. Washington her oral medications: amiodarone 200 mg PO, amlodipine 10 mg PO, and valsartan 320 mg PO. You also must change her nitroglycerine (Nitroderm) patch. You note that her blood pressure is a little high, at 166/88. She complains that she was awake much of the night with a severe headache, so you check to see if she has anything ordered for pain. She has a prn order for Lortab 5 mg for moderate to severe pain. You return to her room about 9:20 a.m. and give her the Lortab. At that time, you also provide a cold cloth for her head, dim the lights, and close the door. At 10:00 a.m., you check back to see how she is feeling. She says the headache is getting better and she thinks she can sleep for a while now.

59. Document the medications you have given on the appropriate place on the medication administration record (MAR; Fig. 35-1). Document any pertinent information on the nurse's note form (Fig. 35-2).

HOSPITAL MEDICATION ADMINISTRATION RECORD

Codes For Injection Sites

A - Left Anterior Thigh	H - Right Anterior Thigh
B - Left Deltoid	I - Right Deltoid
C - Left Gluteus Medius	J - Right Gluteus Medius
D - Left Lateral Thigh	K - Right Lateral Thigh
E - Left Ventral Gluteus	L - Right Ventral Gluteus
F - Left Lower Quadrant	M - Right Lower Quadrant
G - Left Upper Quadrant	N - Right Upper Quadrant

ALLERGIES:				DATE	DATE	DATE
DATE ORDERED	DATE REORD.	DRUG - DOSE - ROUTE - FREQUENCY	ADMIN. TIME			
SIGNATURE / SHIFT INDICATES						
NURSE ADMINISTERING MEDICATIONS						

Figure 35.1 Wilkinson JM, Treas LS: *Fundamentals of Nursing*, Vol 1, 2nd ed., F.A. Davis, Philadelphia, 2011.

| Patient _____ |
| ID# _____ RM _____ |
| BD _____-_____-_____ |
| Admit _____-_____-_____ |
| Physician _____ |

Mission Regional Hospital

Date	Time	Nurse's Notes

Figure 35.2 Nurse's note.

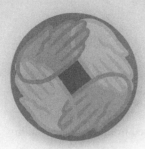

Administering Oral, Topical, and Mucosal Medications

Name: _____

Date: _____

Course: _____

Instructor: _____

Part 1. Key Terms Review

Match the following Key Term(s) or italicized words from your text with the correct description.

_____ 1. Sublingual

_____ 2. Vaginal route

_____ 3. Dry powder inhaler (DPI)

_____ 4. Elixir

_____ 5. Buccal

_____ 6. Metered dose inhaler (MDI)

_____ 7. Solution

_____ 8. Rectal route

_____ 9. Tablet

_____10. Capsule

_____11. Suspension

_____12. Syrup

a. Powdered ingredients pressed into various sizes and shapes

b. Between the cheek and gum

c. Pressurized medication dispensers that spray a premeasured amount of medication

d. Gelatin shell containing a powder or pellets of medication

e. Contains fine particles of medication mixed with but not dissolved in liquid

f. Under the tongue

g. Concentrated aqueous preparation of sugars, with or without flavorings, and medication

h. Administration of creams, suppositories, foams, and tablets into the vagina where they dissolve

i. Contains water, alcohol, possibly colorings, and medication

j. Containers that rely on the force of the patient's own inhalation to dispense a dose of dry powder

k. Administration of suppositories, enemas, ointments, and creams inserted into the rectum

l. A liquid that contains a dissolved substance

Fill in the blank with the correct Key Term(s) or italicized words from your text.

13. The _____ of administration is the method by which medications are taken through the mouth or oral mucous membrane.

14. An _____ tablet contains an outer coating that does not dissolve until the medication reaches the intestines.

15. A _____ tablet is designed to slow the absorption of a drug.

16. When a drug is applied to the skin or mucous membranes, this is administration by the _____.

17. The route used when applying a drug to the skin using a patch is known as the _____ .

18. When medications are dispersed in fine droplets and inhaled into the lungs and bronchial airways, they are administered via the _____.

19. Medications made with opium and opium derivatives for the purpose of controlling and relieving pain are referred to as _____.

Part 2. Connection Questions

Choose the correct answer(s). In some questions, more than one answer is correct. Select all that apply.

20. When you prepare to administer medications through a percutaneous endoscopic gastrostomy (PEG) tube, it is important to determine:
    a. The compatibility of the tube feeding formula with the ordered medications
    b. Whether the medications can be crushed for administration through a PEG
    c. Whether to mix the crushed medications with water or with juice
    d. The brand and length of the PEG tube that is in place

21. You are working in a long-term care facility where certified medication aides administer oral and topical medications. Which of the following concerns you the most?
    a. Ensuring that the medications that you prepare are given by the medication aide
    b. Ensuring that you document all the medications that the aide has administered
    c. Ensuring that all medications are being given correctly
    d. Ensuring that all medication aides are high school graduates

22. You are visiting a client during a home health rotation. The client is having difficulty remembering whether she has taken her medications. What could you do to help this client?
    a. Arrange for her family members to visit her daily to see if she has taken her medications.
    b. Ask a neighbor to call her daily to remind her to take her medications.
    c. Tell her that you will call her daily to remind her to take her medications.
    d. Set up her medications in a pill organizer so she can tell when she has taken them.

23. You are working in a long-term care facility. When will you reorder medications for the resident?
    a. When 7 days remain on the punch card
    b. When 5 days remain on the punch card
    c. When 3 days remain on the punch card
    d. When the punch card is empty

24. You are teaching a patient how to use a metered-dose inhaler (MDI). What information will you include?
    a. Shake the inhaler before using it.
    b. Place the mouthpiece directly into the mouth.
    c. Inhale deeply while depressing the canister.
    d. Hold your breath for 20 seconds.
    e. Breathe out slowly through pursed lips.
    f. Wait 10 seconds before taking the second puff.

25. When teaching how to avoid thrush as a side effect of using a steroid MDI, you would instruct the patient to:
    a. Always use a spacer.
    b. After using the inhaler, rinse his or her mouth with water and spit it out.
    c. Use steroid inhalers before other inhalers.
    d. Clean the mouthpiece in boiling water daily.

26. When you prepare medications for a patient, you learn that she has been taken to the radiology department for an MRI. You administer her medications 2 hours late once she returns to the nursing unit. The patient has blood levels of a seizure medication ordered today. What action will you take?
    a. Notify the physician that the medications were given late.
    b. Complete an incident report because the medications were given more than 1 hour late.
    c. Write an order to omit today's blood draw.
    d. Notify the laboratory of the time that the medications were given and the reason for the delay.

27. You are working in a facility that uses unlicensed personnel to administer medications to adults with developmental disabilities. A newly hired male medication aide seems hesitant when assigned to administer medications on a skilled nursing unit where some residents have PEG tubes. What action will you take?
    a. Say nothing and let him ask questions if he needs help.
    b. Send another medication aide to help him give the medications on that hall.
    c. Ask him to demonstrate giving medications through a PEG tube for you.
    d. Tell him not to give the PEG medications and that you will do it instead.

Part 3. Review Questions

Choose the correct answer(s). In some questions, more than one answer is correct. Select all that apply.

28. Which are included in the oral route of administration?
    a. Swallowing
    b. Sublingual
    c. Inhaling
    d. Buccal
    e. Nasal

29. Which is not a form of oral medications?
    a. Tablets
    b. Creams
    c. Capsules
    d. Liquids

30. If an enteric-coated tablet was crushed and administered through a PEG tube, what would be the result?
    a. The patient would get too much medication at one time, causing an overdose.
    b. The patient would not get the desired effect from the medication because of contact with stomach acid.
    c. The patient would experience gastric irritation because the tablets are not designed to dissolve until they reach the intestines.
    d. The patient would still get the desired effects from the medication with no increase in ill effects.

31. How is a sublingual medication absorbed?
    a. Through numerous blood vessels in the inner cheek
    b. Slowly through the intestinal mucosa
    c. Through the mucous membranes of the nose
    d. Through the numerous blood vessels under the tongue

32. You are preparing to administer a liquid suspension. What must you do first?
    a. Shake the bottle well to mix the medication with the liquid.
    b. Measure the medication and have it checked by another licensed person.
    c. Rotate the bottle carefully between the palms to mix it.
    d. Clean the lid of the bottle with an alcohol swab before opening it.

33. You are pouring a liquid medication. Which actions will you take?
    a. Set the medication cup on top of the medication case and stoop to eye level to pour.
    b. Hold the bottle so the label is in the palm of your hand to avoid spills on the label.
    c. For elderly patients, use a calibrated dropper or syringe to measure the medication.
    d. Measure the amount of liquid in a medication cup at the lowest level of the meniscus.

34. A patient complains of incision pain after surgery. Two pain medications are ordered: Meperidine (Demerol) 75 mg for moderate to severe pain and hydrocodone with acetaminophen (Lortab) 7.5/500 mg for mild to moderate pain. The patient rates her pain at a 5 on a 0 to 10 scale. Her vital signs are T 98.8, P 86, R 14, and BP 104/60. Your next action would be to:
    a. Administer the Demerol prescribed for moderate to severe pain.
    b. Instruct the patient to wait an hour for her pain medication to see if her blood pressure increases.
    c. Administer Lortab prescribed for mild to moderate pain.
    d. Administer 1 dose of Demerol and 1 dose of Lortab together to relieve her pain.

35. What is the preferred way of disposing of oral narcotics that must be wasted?
    a. Crush the extra medication and rinse it down the sink in front of a witness.
    b. Flush the extra medication down the toilet in front of a witness.
    c. Dispose of the extra medication in a chemical waste container in front of a witness.
    d. Place the unused portion of the narcotic back in the narcotic drawer in front of a witness.

36. Why is it necessary to flush a feeding tube with 30 to 60 mL of water before and after administration of medications?
    a. To prevent interactions of medications with the formula in the tube
    b. To give the patient some much-needed fluid intake
    c. To prevent adherence of the drug to the tube
    d. To ensure fluid and electrolyte balance is maintained
    e. To prevent clogging of the tube

37. When you are administering medications to elderly patients, which assessments will you make?
    a. Take a full set of vital signs before administering any medications.
    b. Monitor for increased neurological side effects, toxicity symptoms, and undesired effects frequently.
    c. Assess lung sounds and bowel sounds before administering any medications.
    d. Assess liver and kidney function tests for toxic effects of medications.
    e. Monitor for possible interactions of prescribed and over-the-counter medicines and supplements.

38. How can you be certain that the medication dose for an infant or child is correct before you administer it?
    a. Call the pharmacist each time you administer a medication to confirm the dose.
    b. Double-check the amount of an appropriate pediatric dosage.
    c. Use an oral syringe because it offers more accurate dosing.
    d. Give the child a frozen juice bar before you administer medications.
    e. Have another nurse check the medication dose with you.

39. A patient has an order for silver sulfadiazine (Silvadene) cream to be applied liberally to a burn on the forearm. How will you administer this medication?
    a. Use a tongue depressor to apply a thick coat of medication to the arm.
    b. Use a cotton-tipped applicator to apply a thin covering of medication to the arm.
    c. Place the tip of the medication tube against the burn and squeeze the tube until the burn is covered with the medication.
    d. Apply a thin coat of medication onto a gauze 4 × 4 and place it over the burn.

40. You are teaching a male patient to apply a nitroglycerin transdermal patch. You know the patient needs more teaching when he states:
    a. "I will be sure I remove the previous patch prior to putting on a new one."
    b. "I will put the patch on a place without much body hair."
    c. "I will not cut the patch to make it fit a smaller area."
    d. "I will place the new patch in the same place as the previous one."

41. To administer an eye drop, you will place the drop in the:
    a. Inner canthus of the eye
    b. Outer canthus of the eye
    c. Middle part of the lower conjunctival sac
    d. Middle of the eye, directly onto the pupil

42. How can you prevent eye drops from being absorbed into the bloodstream and causing unwanted systemic effects?
    a. Press your gloved fingertips gently against the lacrimal ducts for a few seconds.
    b. Ensure that the medication is for otic use only.
    c. Instruct the patient to sit or lie very still for 5 to 10 minutes after administration.
    d. Press your gloved fingers at the outer canthus of each eye for 30 seconds.

43. Which of the following will you include when teaching the mother of a 2-year-old how to administer ear drops?
    a. Pull the pinna up and back to straighten the ear canal.
    b. Pull the pinna down and back to straighten the ear canal.
    c. Aim the dropper so the drop rolls down the wall of the canal.
    d. Avoid touching the dropper to the ear to prevent pathogens from entering the bottle of medication.
    e. Have the child remain in position with the affected ear up for at least 10 minutes.

44. Which medication would be administered via the nasal route?
    a. Guaifenesin (Mucinex)
    b. Nicotine (Nicotrol)
    c. Timolol (Timoptic)
    d. Calcitonin (Miacalcin)
    e. Steroids (Rhinocort)

45. Prefilled vaginal applicators are generally used for:
    a. The treatment of localized yeast infections
    b. The treatment of systemic yeast infections
    c. The treatment of vaginitis
    d. The treatment of septicemia
    e. Contraception when containing a spermicide

46. Rectal suppositories are contraindicated in patients with:
    a. High potassium levels
    b. Swollen, inflamed hemorrhoids
    c. Constipation
    d. A recent heart attack

47. A patient is taking an albuterol inhaler as a bronchodilator and a steroid inhaler. You would know more teaching was needed when the patient states:
    a. "I will wait 5 minutes between using the inhalers."
    b. "I will hold the inhalers 1½ to 2 inches away from my mouth to use them."
    c. "I will use the steroid inhaler first, then the albuterol inhaler."
    d. "I will wait 1 full minute between each puff from the inhaler."

48. Number in order the steps to administering a rectal suppository.
    _____ a. Insert the suppository rounded tip first with the index finger on the blunt end.
    _____ b. Instruct the patient to hold the suppository in the rectum as long as possible.
    _____ c. Push the suppository past the internal anal sphincter.
    _____ d. After applying gloves, lubricate the tip of the suppository with water-soluble lubricant.
    _____ e. Position the patient in the left Sims position.

Part 4. Application and Critical Thinking Questions

Write a brief answer to the following questions.

49. You are caring for a patient who has had a CVA. He is able to eat pureed foods but cannot swallow whole pills without getting choked. How will you administer his medications that are in tablet form?

_____

_____

_____

_____

50. You are administering omeprazole (Prilosec) via a PEG tube. Explain how this will be different from administering metoprolol (Lopressor), and list the reason for the differences.

_____

_____

_____

_____

51. List two advantages to administering crushed or liquid medications separately through a feeding tube rather than mixed together in one medicine cup.

_____

_____

_____

_____

Situation Questions

◗ *Scenario: Questions 52 and 53 refer to this scenario.*

You are administering medications to several patients in an acute care setting. It has been a very busy morning and you are in a hurry. After you give a patient a newly ordered pain medication, you see that she is allergic to codeine. When you look it up, you find that the pain medication you administered contained 10 mg codeine.

52. What action will you take first?
    a. Notify the prescriber and explain what happened.
    b. Complete an incident report, following facility policy.
    c. Monitor the patient closely for an allergic reaction and take a set of vital signs.
    d. Take a coworker into the break room and explain what has happened.

53. Which nursing responsibility for administering medications did you omit to cause this error?

_____

_____

_____

_____

Documentation Exercise

You are caring for Dean Odell, a 58-year-old male patient who was admitted on August 11, 2017. His date of birth is 6/6/59. His hospital ID is #9607890. Mr. Odell has an order for digoxin 0.25 mg to be given at 0900 daily. Today is August 12, 2017. You check his digoxin level and find that it is 2.0 ng/mL. When you check his pulse, you count it at 56 beats per minute. You hold the medication and notify the physician. At 0925 you speak with Dr. Marvel by telephone. He gives orders to stop the digoxin 0.25 mg and to give no digoxin for 2 days, then restart it at 0.125 mg daily.

54. Document your actions on the MAR (Fig. 36-1), the nurse's note (Fig. 36-2), and the physician's order form (Fig. 36-3).

HOSPITAL MEDICATION ADMINISTRATION RECORD

Codes For Injection Sites

A - Left Anterior Thigh   H - Right Anterior Thigh
B - Left Deltoid   I - Right Deltoid
C - Left Gluteus Medius   J - Right Gluteus Medius
D - Left Lateral Thigh   K - Right Lateral Thigh
E - Left Ventral Gluteus   L - Right Ventral Gluteus
F - Left Lower Quadrant   M - Right Lower Quadrant
G - Left Upper Quadrant   N - Right Upper Quadrant

ALLERGIES:				DATE	DATE	DATE
DATE ORDERED	DATE REORD.	DRUG - DOSE - ROUTE - FREQUENCY	ADMIN. TIME			
SIGNATURE / SHIFT INDICATES						
NURSE ADMINISTERING MEDICATIONS						

Figure 36.1 Wilkinson JM, Treas LS: *Fundamentals of Nursing,* Vol 1, 2nd ed.,
F.A. Davis, Philadelphia, 2011.

Patient _____		
ID# _____ RM _____		
BD _____-_____-_____		Mission Regional Hospital
Admit _____-_____-_____		
Physician _____		

Date	Time	Nurse's Notes

Figure 36.2 Nurse's note.

Patient Name:	Mission Regional Hospital
ID#	*Physician's Order Sheet*

Date	Orders

Figure 36.3 Physician's order form.

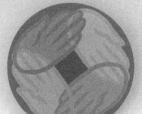

37

Administering Intradermal, Subcutaneous, and Intramuscular Injections

Name: _____

Date: _____

Course: _____

Instructor: _____

Part 1. Key Terms Review

Match the following Key Term(s) or italicized words from your text with the correct description.

_____ 1. Ampule

_____ 2. Gauge

_____ 3. Intradermal

_____ 4. Intramuscular

_____ 5. Subcutaneous

_____ 6. Z-track

_____ 7. Tuberculin syringe

_____ 8. Insulin syringe

_____ 9. Prefilled syringe

_____ 10. Vial

a. Injection technique that closes the needle tract in the tissue, preventing seepage of medication

b. A syringe calibrated in units rather than milliliters

c. Injected into the layers of tissue fat

d. Single-dose, ready-to-use, disposable cartridges

e. Injected directly into the largest portion of a muscle

f. A small, sealed glass drug container that must be broken to withdraw the medication

g. The diameter of the needle, indicated by numbers

h. Inject a small amount of fluid into the dermis

i. Smaller-diameter, 1-mL syringe, calibrated in minims as well as tenths and hundredths of a milliliter; for administering small, precise volumes of medication for infants and TB skin test

j. A glass or plastic container of medication with a rubber stopper that must be punctured with a needle to withdraw medication

Fill in the blank with the correct Key Term(s) or italicized words from your text.

11. The oral route of drug administration results in the drug being routed through the liver, where a portion of the drug is metabolized or used up. This decreases the amount of drug remaining in the blood after it leaves the liver to enter the systemic circulation. This phenomenon is known as _____.

12. One method of decreasing the risk for medication seeping back from the muscle into the subcutaneous tissue along the needle track is to use an _____.

Part 2. Connection Questions

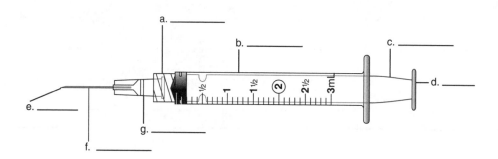

Fill in the blank with the correct labels.

13. Label the parts of the syringe.

(a) _____ (b) _____

(c) _____ (d) _____

14. Label the parts of the needle.

(e) _____ (f) _____

(g) _____

15. How should you dispose of needles?

_____

_____

16. The subcutaneous connective tissue layer contains _____ tissue and larger _____ _____ and _____ .

17. To prevent abscesses and infection of injection sites, you must observe stringent _____ technique while mixing, drawing, and administering injections.

18. For what disease does purified protein derivative (PPD) test? _____

19. How much PPD is administered and what route is it given? _____

20. In which site do you administer a PPD? _____

21. Patients that require repeated insulin injections sometimes develop _____, the breakdown of subcutaneous fat at the site of repeated insulin injections.

22. If the repeated insulin injections at a site caused a buildup of tissue, it is called _____.

Part 3. Review Questions

Choose the correct answer(s). In some questions, more than one answer is correct. Select all that apply.

23. The physician has written an order to administer a PPD to Thomas Staccotti. As you gather your equipment and supplies, you know that you will need which of the following size needles and syringe?
    a. 18 g × 1"
    b. 20 g × $5/_8$"
    c. 25 g × $3/_8$"
    d. 23 g × 1"

24. Some of the following statements regarding insulin are accurate and others are not. Which statement(s) is(are) accurate?
    a. All insulin types can be mixed with other types.
    b. When drawing up regular and intermediate-acting insulins into the same syringe, you must draw the regular insulin first.
    c. Daily injection sites should be rotated once a week.
    d. Insulin is best kept in a dark, dry cabinet.
    e. The preferred site for administering insulin is the back of the upper arm.

25. What gauge and length needle would you select to administer an IM injection of a viscous medication, such as gamma globulin, in the ventrogluteal site of a 29-year-old male body builder who is in good health and weighs 203 pounds?
    a. 25 g × 1.5"
    b. 20 g × $1/_2$"
    c. 21 g × $5/_8$"
    d. 24 g × 1"
    e. 18 g × 1.5"

26. Which of the following sites provides the best and most consistent absorption of insulin?
    a. Upper back
    b. Back of upper arms
    c. Deltoid
    d. Dorsal gluteal
    e. Abdomen

27. Which of the following drugs requires a second and third nurse to verify the dosage?
    a. Insulin
    b. Epinephrine
    c. Heparin
    d. Purified protein derivative

28. What angle of insertion should be used for intradermal injections?
    a. 15 degrees
    b. 30 degrees
    c. 45 degrees
    d. 90 degrees

29. What angle of insertion should be used for intramuscular injections?
    a. 15 degrees
    b. 30 degrees
    c. 45 degrees
    d. 90 degrees

30. What angle of insertion can be used for subcutaneous injections in patients of all sizes?
    a. 15 degrees
    b. 30 degrees
    c. 45 degrees
    d. 90 degrees

31. Which site is the site of choice for IM injections in the majority of patients?
    a. Dorsal gluteal
    b. Deltoid
    c. Ventrogluteal
    d. Vastus lateralis

32. What is the *maximum* volume of medication that can be instilled into the deltoid muscle of the average-size adult?
    a. 3 mL
    b. 2 mL
    c. 1 mL
    d. 0.5 mL
    e. 0.1 mL

33. What is the maximum volume you can instill in the ventrogluteal site of a very large muscular female of approximately 240 pounds?
    a. 3 mL
    b. 2 mL
    c. 1 mL
    d. 0.5 mL
    e. 0.1 mL

34. Which muscle(s)/site(s) is(are) used for injections in infants who are younger than 7 months?
    a. Femoris rectus
    b. Deltoid
    c. Vastus lateralis
    d. Ventrogluteal
    e. Dorsogluteal

35. You would aspirate before injecting the medication in which of the following injections?
    a. 1 mL promethazine IM
    b. 1 mL purified protein derivative ID
    c. Novolin R Insulin 4 units subcut
    d. Heparin 1000 units subcut
    e. Cyanocobalamin 1000 mcg Z-track

36. Which of the following sites would be appropriate to use for an intramuscular injection in a 14-month-old infant with pneumonia?
    a. Femoris rectus
    b. Deltoid
    c. Vastus lateralis
    d. Ventrogluteal
    e. Dorsogluteal

37. You are preparing an intramuscular injection of vitamin K for a newborn who weighs 8 pounds and 8 ounces (3.8 kg). Which of the following needle sizes would be appropriate to use?
    a. 29 g × $^3/_8$"
    b. 25 g × $^5/_8$"
    c. 21 g × 1"
    d. 18 g × 1"
    e. 22 g × 1.5"

Part 4. Application and Critical Thinking Questions

Show all your calculations/work. Then mark the correct syringe by shading in the correct dosage to be drawn up into the syringe.

38. The physician's order reads as follows: *Clindamycin 400 mg IM every 6 hours*.

    The medication label reads: *Clindamycin 155 mg/mL*.

    Which of these syringes would be the most accurate? _____

    How much would you draw into the syringe? _____

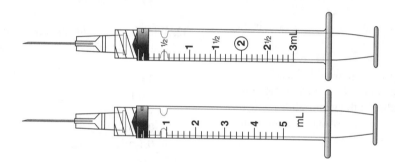

39. The physician's order reads: *Ampicillin 175 mg IM every 6 hours*.

    The medication label reads: *Ampicillin 500 mg/2 mL*.

    Which syringes could you use? _____ and _____

    Which one would be most accurate? _____

    How much will you draw into the syringe? _____

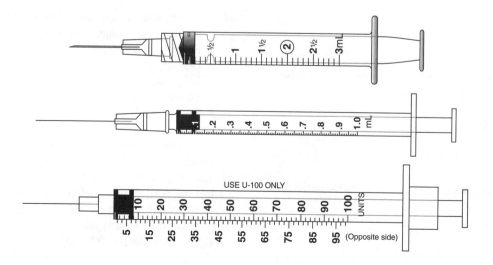

40. The physician's order reads: *Codeine 60 mg IM every 4–6 hr PRN pain.*

    The medication label reads: *Codeine 1 gr/mL.*

    Which syringe will you use? _____

    How much will you draw into the syringe? _____

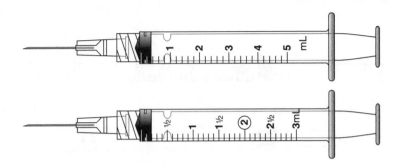

41. The physician's order reads: *NPH Insulin 22 units subcut daily at 0700.*

    The medication label reads: *NPH Insulin U-100/mL.*

    Which syringe will you use? _____

    How much will you draw into the syringe? _____

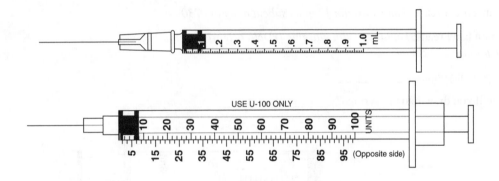

42. The physician's order reads: *Heparin 15,000 units subcut every 12 hours.*

    The medication label reads: *Heparin 20,000 units per mL.*

    Which syringe will you use? _____

    How much will you draw into the syringe? _____

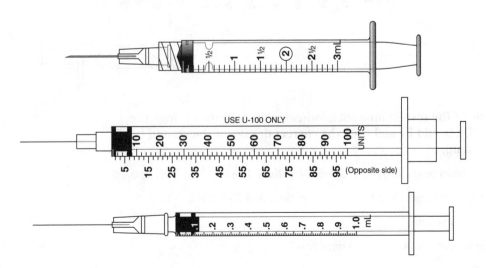

43. The physician's order reads: *PPD 0.1 mL ID today.*

    The medication label reads: *Tubersol-Tuberculin Purified Protein Derivative, 5 U.S. units per test dose (0.1 mL).*

    Which syringe will you use? _____

    How much will you draw into the syringe? _____

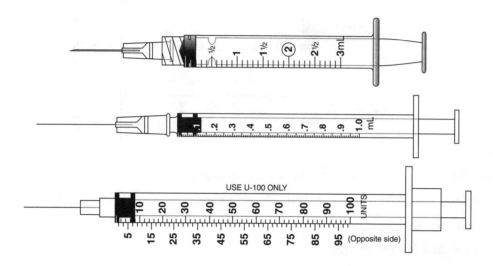

44. The physician's order reads: *Lantus insulin 17 units subcut daily at 0730.*

    The medication label reads: *Lantus (insulin glargine [rDNA origin] injection) solution for subcutaneous injection.*

    Which syringe will you use? _____

    How much will you draw into the syringe? _____

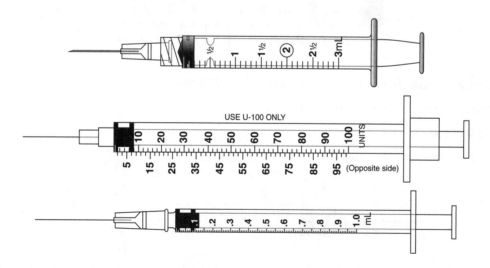

When you shade in the insulin amounts, indicate where in the syringe the first drawn insulin would be and then the correct dosage of the second insulin to be drawn up.

45. The physician's order reads: *NPH 12 units and Novolin R 3 units subcut daily at 0700.*

    The medication labels read: *NPH U-100/mL and Novolin R U-100/mL.*

    Which syringe will you use? _____

    Which insulin will you draw into the syringe first? _____

How much of each insulin will you draw into the syringe? _____

What will be the total volume of insulin in the syringe after both are drawn up?
_____

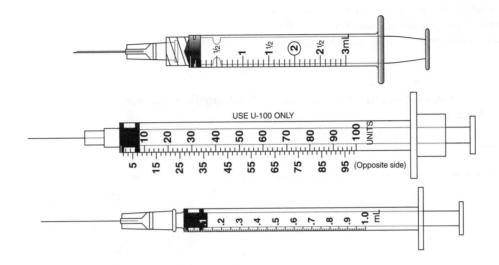

46. The physician's order reads: *Lantus 10 units with Regular 4 units subcut now.*

    What is the problem with this insulin order? _____

Situation Questions

▶ *Scenario: Question 47 refers to this scenario.*

Your patient's name is Melissa Hall. She is in Room 307 and her hospital ID is #3411576. Her BD is March 1, 1966. She was admitted on August 19, 2017. Today's date is August 20, 2017, and it is 0135.

   Ms. Hall is crying and complaining of abdominal pain in the vicinity of her surgical incision. She reports that it is severe—an 8 on a scale of 0 to 10. The characteristics are sharp and stabbing, worsening whenever she moves. She tells you that she is not nauseated at this time. She has a physician's order for Stadol 2 mg IM every 4 hours prn for pain. Her last dose was at 2017. At 0145, not only do you administer the analgesic in her right ventrogluteal site, but you also decide to implement some nonpharmaceutical measures to make her more comfortable. You massage her back with lotion after repositioning her on the right side. You provide her with a cup of hot cocoa, which she drinks. At 0215 you assess Ms. Hall for the effectiveness of the interventions. She reports that her pain in now a 4 and that she is getting sleepy.

47. Use a nurse's note form (Fig. 37-1) and narrative-style documentation to document this scenario.

Write a brief answer to the following question.

▸ *Scenario: Question 48 refers to this scenario.*

You are to administer a 1-mL intramuscular injection to a 94-year-old female who weighs just under 100 pounds (45.4 kg). She is frail and emaciated. You plan to administer the injection in her ventrogluteal site in the gluteus medius.

48. Besides the medication, what supplies should you gather? What specific needle size and length will you use?

_____

_____

Patient _____		Mission Regional Hospital
ID# _____ RM _____		
BD _____-_____-_____		
Admit _____-_____-_____		
Physician _____		

Date	Time	Nurse's Notes

Figure 37.1 Nurse's note.

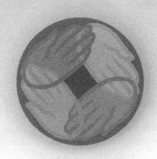

Peripheral IV Therapy

Name:	
Date:	
Course:	
Instructor:	

Part 1. Key Terms Review

Match the following Key Term(s) or italicized words from your text with the correct description.

_____ 1. Isotonic

_____ 2. Cannulation

_____ 3. Patent

_____ 4. Nonvesicant

_____ 5. Hypotonic

_____ 6. Hemolysis

_____ 7. Infiltration

_____ 8. Hypertonic

_____ 9. Hypovolemia

_____ 10. Parenteral

a. Solution has a lower osmolarity than body fluids

b. Type of medicine that does not cause blistering and death of tissue on infiltration

c. Lysis or destruction of RBCs

d. Infusion of fluids, electrolytes, and nutritional components by a route other than the usual route of the alimentary canal

e. The decrease in blood volume when fluids and electrolytes are lost in balanced proportions from extracellular spaces

f. Leakage of nonvesicant IV fluid or medication into the tissue surrounding the IV insertion site

g. The process of advancing the IV cannula into the vein

h. A fluid that has a higher concentration of particles dissolved in it than fluids of the body

i. Open

j. Fluid that contains an amount of solute that produces a concentration of dissolved particles equal to that of the intracellular and extracellular fluids of the human body

Fill in the blank with the correct Key Term(s) or italicized words from your text.

11. The word that means similar to infiltration but involves leakage of vesicant IV fluid medication into the tissue surrounding the IV insertion site is known as

    _____.

12. The liquid portion of the blood is known as

    _____.

13. The plastic projection that provides a place for your fingers to push the piercing pin into the solution bag port without contaminating the sterile piercing pin is known as the _____.

14. In reference to the blood vessels, a word that means hardened is _____.

15. A _____ forms when one of the agents in a solution separates from the solvent and becomes a solid, insoluble product that looks cloudy, hazy, or like fine floating crystals.

16. _____ refers to a type of medication that causes blistering, necrosis, and sloughing of tissue when allowed to enter the subcutaneous tissue.

17. The interaction between the two drugs that causes a change in the activity or components of one or more of the drugs is known as a _____.

18. The red blood cells that have been separated from plasma for transfusion are called _____.

19. Another term for blood clot is _____.

Part 2. Connection Questions

Choose the correct answer(s). In some questions, more than one answer is correct. Select all that apply.

20. Before you can safely administer IV medications, there are several things that you must know including:
    a. If the patient has ever had IV medications before
    b. Patient's medication allergies
    c. Patient's disease or condition
    d. Sterile technique

21. When you are administering hypotonic IV fluids, you know that the fluids are going to:
    a. Cause shifting of body fluids into the intravascular space
    b. Cause shifting of body fluids from the intracellular spaces into the interstitial spaces
    c. Cause shifting of body fluids out of the intravascular space and into the interstitial spaces, and then eventually into the intracellular spaces, rehydrating the cells
    d. Remain in their original fluid compartments

22. Because of the fluid shifts in the previous question, prolonged infusion of this type fluid when it is not needed can result in which of the following?
    a. Cerebral cells swelling
    b. Increased intracranial pressure
    c. Dehydration of cells
    d. Edema

23. Which fluid is best when an individual needs only simple water replacement because of lack of fluid intake or loss of body water without loss of electrolytes, known as hypertonic dehydration?
    a. Isotonic fluid
    b. Hypotonic fluid
    c. Hypertonic fluid

24. Which type IV fluid will cause cellular dehydration if infused unnecessarily?
    a. Isotonic fluid
    b. Hypotonic fluid
    c. Hypertonic fluid

25. Which of the following IV catheters with plastic cannulas are the smallest in diameter?
    a. 16 g
    b. 18 g
    c. 21 g
    d. 25 g
    e. 29 g

26. You are about to attempt to initiate an IV on a 97-year-old female with tiny, fragile veins. Which of the following access devices would most likely be your best choice?
    a. 27 g × 1" winged butterfly without cannula
    b. 22 g × 1 ¼" Intracath
    c. 25 g × 1" winged butterfly with cannula
    d. 23 g × 1" Intracath

27. How does an intermittent prn lock differ from a traditional IV site?
    a. The prn lock is used for continual infusion of IV fluids or medications.
    b. The patient with a prn lock must be stuck each time medication needs to be administered.
    c. The prn lock provides subcutaneous access rather than IV access.
    d. The prn lock allows for intermittent infusion of IV fluids or medications without requiring a continual infusion of fluids.

28. Which of the following explanations of the differences between IV push and IVPB routes of administration are correct?
    a. The IV push route of administration allows direct infusion from the bag of solution at a rapid rate, which pushes the medication in quickly.
    b. The IVPB route of administration allows medications to infuse over a 1- to 2-minute interval.
    c. The IVPB route of administration requires that the medication be dissolved in a volume of fluid, ranging between 50 and 250 mL.
    d. The IV push route of administration provides for direct injection of medication into the port closest to the IV site.

29. Which of the following is the most important concept related to IV therapy?
    a. Maintain strict asepsis.
    b. Monitor IV infusion rate.
    c. Maintain fluid balance.
    d. Educate the patient about the IV therapy.

Part 3. Review Questions

Match each IV fluid with the appropriate term that accurately describes the fluid's tonicity.

30. _____ 0.45% NS

31. _____ D5½NS

32. _____ ⅓NS

33. _____ 0.9% NS

34. _____ D5W

35. _____ LR

36. _____ D5¼NS

37. _____ Normosol R

38. _____ D5 NS

a. Isotonic
b. Hypotonic
c. Hypertonic

Part 4. Application and Critical Thinking Questions

Choose the correct answer(s). In some questions, more than one answer is correct. Select all that apply.

39. Which of the following rates would be considered to be a "keep the vein open" rate?
    a. 30 mL/hr
    b. 75 mL/hr
    c. 80 mL/hr
    d. 100 mL/hr

40. Which of the following should be assessed prior to initiating an IV?
    a. Toughness of the patient's skin
    b. Purpose of the IV
    c. If allergic to tape, latex, or iodine
    d. The patient's white blood cell count results

41. You are preparing the supplies to initiate an IV for one of your patients. You have assessed the expiration date of the IV tubing package and removed it from the packaging. Which of the following should you perform prior to spiking the IV solution bag?
    a. Close the roller clamp on the tubing.
    b. Prepare the IV start kit for use.
    c. Label the solution bag.
    d. Ensure that the air has been removed from the tubing.

42. Which of the following restrictions is(are) accurate with regard to selecting a vein for use when restarting an infiltrated IV?
    a. You cannot use the same vein again for 12 hours.
    b. You should use the same arm again to prevent soreness in both of the patient's arms.
    c. If you use the same vein where the IV infiltrated, you must use a site distal to the old site.
    d. The best veins to use are those of the forearm.
    e. Once an IV has infiltrated in the forearm, it should be restarted in the hand on that arm.

43. Characteristics of a "good" vein site to use for IV initiation include which of the following?
    a. Vein feels firm, hard, and sturdy
    b. Vein has a bifurcation
    c. Vein feels spongy and bouncy
    d. Vein rolls easily
    e. Vein is easy to feel

Write a brief answer to the following questions.

44. Which of the following vascular access devices is(are) commonly used for scalp veins in newborns? _____

45. What is the term for removing air from the IV tubing? _____

46. Name four of the most commonly used veins for IV initiation. _____

_____

_____

47. The physician has ordered the IV to infuse at 100 mL/hr. The tubing's drop factor is 12. Calculate the gravity infusion rate. Show your work. _____

_____

_____

48. The physician has ordered the IV to infuse at 75 mL/hr. The tubing's drop factor is 10. Calculate the gravity infusion rate. Show your work. _____

_____

_____

49. The physician has ordered the IV to infuse at 125 mL/hr. The tubing's drop factor is 20. Calculate the gravity infusion rate. Show your work. _____

_____

_____

50. The physician has ordered the IV to infuse at 30 mL/hr. The tubing's drop factor is 60. Calculate the gravity infusion rate. Show your work. _____

_____

_____

51. The IVPB is to infuse over 30 minutes. The PB solution bag is 50 mL. The tubing's drop factor is 12. Calculate the gravity infusion rate. Show your work.

_____

_____

52. The IVPB is to infuse over 30 minutes. The PB solution bag is 100 mL. The tubing's drop factor is 20. Calculate the gravity infusion rate. Show your work.

_____

_____

53. The IVPB is to infuse over 20 minutes. The PB solution bag is 100 mL. The tubing's drop factor is 20. Calculate the gravity infusion rate. Show your work.

_____

_____

Documentation Exercise

▶ *Scenario:*

The patient in Room 500 is Shandy Baggs. She was admitted on 7/10/17. Her birth date is 4/22/76. Her hospital ID is #668899. Today's date is 7/10/17, and it is 1325. You just finished initiating an IV in her right forearm. It took you three sticks. You finally got a 22-gauge Intracath in. You started 1000 mL of D51/2NS with the additive 40 mEq KCL. It is infusing via an IV pump at 80 mL/hr as ordered. She denies any discomfort.

54. Use a nurse's note form (Fig. 38-1) and narrative-style documentation to document this scenario.

Patient _____
ID# _____ RM _____
BD _____-_____-_____
Admit _____-_____-_____
Physician _____

Mission Regional Hospital

Date	Time	Nurse's Notes

Figure 38.1 Nurse's note.

Illustration Credits